THE BODY'S "ACUPUNCTURE" ENERGETICS

THE BODY'S "ACUPUNCTURE" ENERGETICS

Henry Gacrama dela Torre, M.D.

Fellow, American Academy of Medical Acupuncture

Copyright © 2010 by Henry Dela Torre.

Library of Congress Control Number: 2010917045
ISBN: Hardcover   978-1-4568-1679-7
               Softcover   978-1-4568-1678-0
               Ebook   978-1-4568-1680-3

All rights reserved. No part of this book may be reproduced or transmitted in any form or by any means, electronic or mechanical, including photocopying, recording, or by any information storage and retrieval system, without permission in writing from the copyright owner.

This book was printed in the United States of America.

To order additional copies of this book, contact:
Xlibris Corporation
1-888-795-4274
www.Xlibris.com
Orders@Xlibris.com
88158

CONTENTS

Introduction ix

Chapter I	God's Creation	1
Chapter II	The Beginning of Time	4
Chapter III	The Three Basic Energies of the Body (According to Chinese teachings)	9
Chapter IV	Yuan Qi Genetic Energy	13
Chapter V	Rong Qi Nutritional Energy	17
Chapter VI	Wei Qi Controlling Energy	29
Chapter VII	The Body's Energetic Flow	33
Chapter VIII	Yin and Yang Concepts	37
Chapter IX	Yang Excess Syndrome	43
Chapter X	Yin Deficiency Syndrome	45
Chapter XI	Heat Illnesses and Cold Illnesses	47
Chapter XII	The Role of Emotions in our Health: The Five Element Acupuncture Energetics	50
Chapter XIII	Energetic Personalities Structural Biopsychotypes	55
Chapter XIV	Body, Mind, and Soul	63
Chapter XV	Flash Signs and Symptoms	67
Chapter XVI	Taking Charge of One's Health: The Body Systems	70
Chapter XVII	Maintenance of Normal Body Temperature	90
Chapter XVIII	Hair Function	93
Chapter XIX	Sexual Function/Activity	95
Chapter XX	Water Balance	99

Chapter XXI	The Ten Commandments of Health	102
Chapter XXII	Sins Against the Body and Nature	105
Chapter XXIII	The Triad	109
Chapter XXIV	Energetic Massage: Early Healing of Acute Medical Problems	111
Chapter XXV	The Conclusion	115

About the Author 121
Bibliography 123
Index 127

DEDICATION

I would like to dedicate this book to my lovely wife, Elvie, and our four lovely daughters, Crystal Ann, Liz Abegail, Vanessa, and Roseanne. I thank them for all their support and for allowing me to practice my acupuncture knowledge on them. I thank my mentors, especially Dr. Joseph Helms and his staff who taught me acupuncture. I also thank all my patients for the privilege of treating them with acupuncture and all patients who have taught me valuable lessons from their illnesses. I hope this book will help a lot of people to take better care of their health.

INTRODUCTION

The human body has been amazingly created by a "Supreme Being" whom most of us call, God. Many people call "The Supreme Being" many names but I will call God in this book.

God created the human body from the beginning of creation and providing it with all the means necessary to grow, heal, and survive in this world. Our creation and existence in this world is but a test of some higher purpose. But for us to succeed, He implanted in each one of us the seed for growth, function, and healing. He implanted in us the ability to assimilate food and grow as well as perform unimaginable physical and mental activities. He implanted in us the ability to perform analyses, deductions, and decisions. He implanted in our body the defense mechanisms necessary to protect our bodies from the outside forces of nature that are harmful to us. He also implanted in each one of us the tremendous healing power to repair our bodies after an injury or illness. He gave us emotions in order to allow us to interact with each other as part of our test in this life. All the natural things around us exist for a reason, which in the long run, is possibly to help us accomplish our ultimate purpose in this life.

All the animals, trees, and plants around us exist for three reasons, as God gave them to us. They are for nutrition, healing, and beauty. I am not quite sure why certain animals and plants are poisonous to mankind, except that God puts them in these God's creations to protect them from other predators.

Plants and animals around us were put in this world to sustain our nourishment in order to give us energy and be able to perform all activities necessary for our survival. These activities are farming, fishing, harvesting, gathering of food, making and fixing our dwellings to protect us from the elements, as well as taking care of other God's creations, which include the human race as well as the animal and plant kingdoms.

Similarly, God put into this world certain plants for medicinal purposes or to promote health and/or healing. It is not surprising, therefore, that a lot of plants are utilized by different cultures for healing, whether on its own or in combination. Some of these medicinal plants are aloe vera, goji, mangosteen, ginseng, astragalus, ginger, milk thistle, cinnamon, apricot, the coconut, and countless other fruits and plants.

Other plants and trees that don't have nutritional or medicinal properties are generally endowed with beauty. They, therefore, derive their healing properties through the soul or spirit. It calms the soul, and it relaxes the mind, which is an integral part to a healthy body and to our well-being. Beautiful trees, plants, flowers, animals, birds, and fishes function to enhance our experience in this life and give us excitement and fulfillment. They are not to be consumed but to be enjoyed. They function as enhancements to this journey in life.

It is my hope that this book will help not only medical practitioners, but also laypeople. This book aims to simplify the human body and how it functions, going down to the basic physical and energetic functions of the body. I hope that through this book all people will realize that the primary responsibility of our health maintenance solely rests upon each one of us. Patients should not relinquish that responsibility to others, including to healing practitioners.

CHAPTER I

God's Creation

It is my belief that God created us for a reason, which to me, is to ultimately join Him in heaven.

According to the bible, when God created the first angel, Lucifer, God endowed him with some of his powers. He was created to the likeness of God, therefore, he had characteristics similar to God. He had healing powers (self-healing), power to generate energy, the power to think and speak, perform multitude of things, and other capabilities that Lucifer thought he could also be a God. Therefore, he was banished by God to hell. This probably prompted God to decide to test His "angels" first before admitting them into heaven. This He did after the three Archangels, Michael, Gabriel and Raphael were created. Thus, God created the universe in six days. These creations (the sun and moon, the oceans, land, plants, and animals) were made for the single purpose of providing for His **angels** who are to be on trial before being admitted into heaven. We are His angels, but before He can try us, He had to provide us with the light, the energy, as well as the place to stay. He also provided us the sustenance needed in order to stay alive, grow, and propagate. Thus God created the universe, especially the sun, the earth and the moon in order to provide us with the light, energy as well as the place to stay.

The sun's energy provides sunlight to the plants for them to process food, grow, and multiply. God provided the plants and trees three things in order to survive, namely, the earth with its nutrients, water, and carbon dioxide. Water and nutrients are absorbed from the earth and with the action of the sunlight, these are processed into food by the plants and trees by the process of photosynthesis. As a result, oxygen is released as by-product to be used by humans and animals for metabolism. After humans have utilized the oxygen for their own metabolism, we then exhale carbon dioxide (CO2), which is absorbed by the plants through their leaves. Plants serve as our filters, splitting CO2 into carbon which plants utilize for food and release the Oxygen which man utilize for metabolism. Carbon from decaying plants and animals is absorbed by the earth to absorb heat from the sun and ultimately converted into energy for us. This will be in the form of fossil fuels like oil, gas and coal. This will then repeat the cycle.

We indirectly derive energy from the sun by eating the plants around us as well as the animals and fish nourished by these plants. We likewise derive direct energy from the sun through the activation of our hypothalamus-pituitary axis, stimulating it to produce the Adrenocorticotrophic hormones (ACTH) in order to wake us up, provide us with the energy to perform our various tasks, as well as protect us from injury and death through our "fright and flight" reflex. This reflex is mainly controlled by our adrenal gland by releasing adrenaline and giving us the energy to run or defend ourselves.

The sun even helps us produce melatonin to help us sleep and produce vitamin D, a very important vitamin for our structure, the musculoskeletal system. In acupuncture sense, the energy of the sun is absorbed by our body and moves the nutritional energy in our body by stimulating the circulation of the blood and also creating a zone of energy flow around us which the Chinese call Wei Qi, which I call **Protective energy**.

God decided to place us on earth to stay, interact among each other, and to propagate the human race. We have to appreciate the purpose of our lives and all the things God has provided us in order to survive. For in understanding the mechanics for which God has intended our bodies to function, be sustained, and how we protect ourselves from disease and harm, can we then better take care of our bodies and ultimately not only the human race but this world as well? We just have to remember that the **rule of nature** which governs our existence is inseparable from its Creator, God.

CHAPTER II

The Beginning of Time

God first created the sun and the moon for a reason. The sun controls our **biorhythm**. It also indirectly controls our nutrition, growth, and healing process. By rotating the earth along its axis, it assures us that we get our fair share of the sunlight. After all, it is the sun that wakes us up in the morning. It is accomplished by the radiation of the sun's rays like the ultraviolet rays and other rays, which trigger the release of pituitary hormones, especially the Adrenocorticotrophic hormone (ACTH), growth hormone, and ultimately cortisol, and the adrenomedullary hormone, adrenalines. Both cortisol and adrenaline are in highest concentration in the early morning.

By the action of the sun's ultraviolet rays and electromagnetic forces, these rays trigger the pituitary gland to release ACTH which stimulates the adrenal glands to release cortisol. Adrenaline is likewise released by the Sympathetic system. These are our "starters," similar to the car starter motor. It wakes us up and primes us to get up and start working. It is, therefore, important that we get up as soon as we wake up at sunrise, or our body will go into an "idling" mode. Like the car, "idling" the engine causes overheating. Staying in bed after sunrise tends to overheat the body also. It is, therefore, not surprising that people who get up late in the morning, when the sun is already way up on the horizon (past 9:00 a.m.), tend to develop heat problems and pain problems, namely, headache, chronic pain or even gastrointestinal problems like irritable bowel syndrome or colitis, and they also have no energy.

With sunrise, we wake up and our day starts. This is the beginning in the flow of the Nutritional Energy. Of foremost importance is the stomach energy since it is the channel that provides the primary energy that is distributed to all the body organs. It is this energy derived from food that we call **Nutritional Energy** that powers the different body organs to function. It is not unusual that we wake up with the sunrise, and if we don't get up, then we have a tendency to wake up every thirty to sixty minutes or so, as well as dream while trying to sleep. This is because our "starters", the adrenal glands are beating us up with minute releases of these hormones at regular intervals. And if we don't get up until past 9:00 a.m., our levels for these hormones are already depleted so that we have no stamina and no "energy" to perform things until later when the adrenals have recovered and formed enough hormones for us to function. Besides, if we get up way past sunrise, we will have missed out on water (fluids) and food (energy that the brain needs). Therefore, the body becomes weak and overheated. This also causes the person to sleep late, and then the cycle is perpetuated: late bedtime, late getting up, and missing breakfast and fluids.

The flow of Nutritional Energy starts in the stomach. It is said that the **stomach energy** works best between seven and nine in the morning. It is very important, therefore, to eat breakfast in order to provide the body with the necessary energy to be passed around from organ to organ. The saying that "breakfast is the most important meal of the day" probably started from the beginning of time. The energy we get from breakfast will allow the organs of the body to function optimally or what I call the **maximum functional time**. The flow of this Nutritional Energy is maximum in an organ for two hours to maximize its function as the organ is nourished by the nutritional energy. However, twelve hours later, that will also be the time that the organ has its least activity lasting for two hours, or its **resting period**.

That flow of Nutritional Energy may constitute what we know as "biorhythm." Health is, therefore, very dependent in our ability to function according to our biorhythm. Energy generation starts in the morning. It is then that the different organs of the body start functioning in a daytime mood. Failure to follow our biorhythm results in a poorly functioning body, causing fatigue and lack of energy, which may result in illness after a prolong period of time. The result is the body being weakened, unable to protect against the invasion of microorganisms, heat, cold, humidity, wind and radiation.

The Stomach Channel (with maximum energy between 7-9 am) has to receive nutrition for it to be able to provide energy to the body. After the stimulation of the stomach, then the Spleen Channel is activated (pancreas) to help digest the food. The Heart Channel (11:00-1:00 p.m.) is stimulated next in order to pump blood and increase the circulation of blood into the gastrointestinal tract (that carries the nutrients and oxygen). The Small Intestine channel is stimulated next in order to absorb nutrients from the digestive tract. The Bladder Channel (3:00-5:00 p.m.) is increased next, strengthening the back and at the same time helps empty the bladder in preparation for the increased kidney action, and, therefore, increases urinary excretion. After the bladder channel receives its maximum energy, the Kidney Channel follows (5:00-7:00 p.m.). Following the Kidney channel, the following channels will have their maximum activities of two hours each channel: Master of the Heart or Pericardium (7:00-9:00 p.m.); Triple Heater or Triple Burner (9:00-11:00 p.m.); Gallbladder Channel (11:00-1:00 a.m.); the Liver Channel (1:00-3:00 a.m.); Lung Channel (3:00-5:00 a.m.); and finally the Large Intestine Channel (5:00-7:00 a.m.). Then the cycle starts over again the following day.

The Liver Channel takes care of sleep. The liver organ is also involved with detoxification and is probably the major organ involved with the healing process. It has its maximum activity between 1:00 a.m. and 3:00 a.m. It is also responsible for controlling the eyes and feet. It is, therefore, imperative that we should be asleep before this time. Is it possible that REM sleep (rapid eye movement) occurs the most at this time? Is it possible that healing occurs mostly at this time also? People with liver problems like hepatitis, generally wake up between 1:00 a.m. and 3:00 a.m., or they may have problem sleeping. They could either have difficulty sleeping or staying asleep, or they sleep a lot so that once these patients start sleeping through between 1:00-3:00 a.m., then we can use it as an indication of improvement of their liver function.

The Lung Channel is most active between 3:00 a.m. and 5:00 a.m. It is probably the reason that people with asthma have a tendency to have attacks early in the morning. People who have lung problems generally wake up between 3:00 a.m. and 5:00 a.m. Once these patients sleep through the night and into the morning, then we know that their lung condition has improved. Knowing the time of maximum activity of any organ can be of use to determine the improvement of an illness or the prognosis of a patient or a condition.

The Large Intestine Channel is the next channel and is most active between 5:00 a.m. and 7:00 a.m. It is also the reason that most people move their bowels early in the morning as soon as they get up. So, regular bowel movements every morning indicate a good functioning Nutritional Energy, therefore, an indication of good health for the moment. The Stomach Channel (Earth element) in the five element energetic movement is the element that generates energy for the Large Intestine Channel (Metal element). It is, therefore, usual that the large intestine will move (bowel movement) after a meal, the so-called "gastrocolic reflex."

The Stomach Channel is next in the energetic movement of Rong Qi. It is most active between 7:00 a.m. and 9:00 a.m. This is probably the beginning of the cycle for the day. The resulting cortisol release is powerful enough that it wakes us up from our sleep. Cortisol and adrenaline are two adrenal hormones that are powerful enough that doctors utilize them "to bring people from the dead." In other words, physicians use them in "resuscitating the patient whose heart just stopped in cases of cardiac arrest." This is because the kidney channel or adrenal gland controls the heart. We, therefore, use corticosteroids and adrenaline in conjunction with calcium (the mineral that acts as our connection to the earth) to resuscitate people whose heart just stopped. Is it possible that the minerals carbon (main component of our body), calcium (main component of bones) and iron (major component of blood) are responsible for us being grounded to earth?

CHAPTER III

The Three Basic Energies of the Body

(According to Chinese teachings)

There are three basic energies that control the body. They are *Original energy (Yuan Qi), Nutritional energy (Rong Qi), and Controlling energy (Wei Qi)*.

Our "**Original Energy**" (Yuan Qi) is derived from both parents, which is the genetic makeup of an individual (genes or chromosomes). We can call this also our **"Genetic Energy"**. Since it is the chromosomes in our body, we, therefore, have little control over this, although we may be able to enhance it or protect ourselves from its ill effects. Hence, we closely mimic our parents and close relatives. Whatever talents and characteristics that our parents and relatives have, we most likely will get them as well. Unfortunately, whatever illnesses or deficiencies our parents or ancestors have, we likewise would most likely get them. We are what our parents are. Little can be done with any genetic abnormalities. Science, however, may someday find a way of tinkering with genetics as are being done in some illnesses using stem cells. We can, however, mitigate bad genetic influences by following healthy habits or leading a "healthy" lifestyle. God probably bestowed life on us by "breathing" Yuan Qi on us.

Our **Original Energy** (Yuan Qi) resides in the adrenal glands. It is the "battery" of our body that determines our life span. It is of course controlled by the brain through the pituitary gland-hypothalamus axis. We probably have approximately the same life span, but whether we get there or not depend on how we carry out our lifestyles and take care of ourselves. It is, therefore, necessary that we allow the full development of our organs before we utilize them fully, especially the **reproductive organs**. Abusing our adrenals through stress, overindulgence (too much sex, food, and sleep), substance abuse (chemicals, drugs, alcohol, and tobacco products), and inactivity results in **adrenal burnout**. Inactivity in the form of too much sitting, riding vehicles, watching TV or doing computers, typing, writing, and reading, prevents the adrenal glands from functioning properly and from renewing.

Nutritional Energy (Rong Qi) on the other hand is the energy we derive from food. This is the energy that God indirectly provided us through the plants and animals we eat. He provided us the plants, nurtured them with the sun in the presence of water and the nutrients provided by the earth and the sea and with the carbon dioxide provided through man and animals. Our **Controlling Energy** (Wei Qi) is the energy that nurtures us to allow us to grow, heal and repair the body. The stomach and spleen channels (pancreas) are the main controllers of this energy, in conjunction with the heart.

Controlling Energy (Wei Qi) is the energy we derive from the sun, probably mediated by Vitamin D. This is the energy that moves our Nutritional Energy around the body. This we can also call Defensive Energy. This energy envelops the body and rotates around the body during the day so many times. This movement is not the same for all individuals. At night, this energy goes inside the body and into the liver. The Controlling Energy (Wei Qi) comes out from the liver through the eyes, opening our eyes for the day. The inability of this energy to go inside the body and into the liver at night results in insomnia. Similarly, the inability of the Wei Qi to come out through our eyes in the morning results in sleepiness or difficulty in opening our eyes and to get up. That is why people with liver problems will have sleep problems. I don't think our Controlling Energy revolves around our body at a fixed rate. I also believe that **there are three Controlling Energies that surround our body**. Just as there are three influences that affect the oceans, there are also three Controlling Energies that control us.

The first energy is analogous to the effect of the moon on the ocean, as well as on humans. Just as the moon affects the tide of the ocean, the moon also affects a person's *mood*. This is due to our sodium chloride content in the body which is analogous to the ocean. The first Controlling Energy, I will call the **Energy Pool** (Major Wei Qi). This is the energy that we directly receive from the sun, and indirectly through the moon. This effect is slow but tremendous, more noticeable in certain individuals with weaknesses in their Controlling energy. Since this energy affects our general overall energy and mood, this is responsible for our "bipolarity". All human beings have bipolarities; but normally, we cycle from happiness (mania) to depression infrequently and less extreme. Most people will cycle slowly and with little fluctuations. However, some people will cycle at extremes, or stay in one end of the spectrum more than the other end. So, we see people who are "manic" and we see people who are depressed. We also see people who cycle fast at the extreme ends (mania and depression) and we classify them as bipolar. These are just nothing more but modulations of our "Energy Pool". Our Energy Pool does not flow, but is the source of our Controlling energy (Wei Qi). It gives rise to the Protective energy.

The second Controlling Energy (Wei Qi) is a large wave that mainly carries the flow of the energy around the body from one energetic channel to another. This energy is derived from the "Energy Pool" and is responsible for moving the Nutritional Energy (Rong Qi). This I call, the **Protective Energy** (Wei Qi). This gives the strength and stamina of an individual, provides healing from trauma and disease as well as protects us from trauma. I felt my Protective energy before which does not correspond to my heart beat, flowed along my Small Intestine channel and rotates around the body around 30 times per minute. This energy flow varies from individual to individual, and the strength or force, as well as its speed of flow, determines the efficiency of the Protective energy as well as the strength of an individual. This varies from time to time as well, depending on the nutritional status, water content of the body, outside temperature and or presence of obstruction in the channel. The Protective energy protects us from outside energy invasion, such heat, wind, cold, humidity, radiation and other outside forces.

The third Controlling energy (Wei Qi) is smaller but moves faster than the Protective energy. This corresponds to the surface waves in the sea. This energy is the residual energy from the Protective energy, usually in the form of sweat. This protects us from microorganisms by creating an electrical charge on the surface of the body. This I call **Electrostatic Energy**, or Minor Wei Qi. This is especially strong when we are perspiring since the resulting sodium chloride released causes the electromagnetic charge which traps and "electrocutes" microorganisms.

CHAPTER IV

Yuan Qi

Genetic Energy

"**G**enetic Energy" is the **Original Energy**, the source of all energies. The Chinese calls it Yuan Qi. It is the energy passed on to us from our parents. It represents our genetic makeup, our chromosomes passed on to us from our mother's egg, and our father's sperm. From these two cells, its union results in the formation of a fetus that is nourished by the mother and comes out almost exactly nine months later into a complete being with its parts in exactly a predetermined location and function. Hence, the eyes are always on the face, on each side with the nose in front and with all the different organs of the body in exactly the same location. The functions of the different organs are also the same among all individuals. This is so because God placed in our bodies the **memory chip** for each cell to develop into tissues and organs with specific functions. These tissues and organs are derived from "stem cells" or original cells, the precursors of all cells and tissues. But fortunately, since these organs are derived from the same set of cells (stem cells), there is, therefore, this connection between all the parts of the body. It is this "energetic connection" between each part of the body that we tap in order to effect change during acupuncture treatments.

However, since Genetic Energy refers to the genetic makeup of the person, we cannot change it much. Our genes or chromosomes were predetermined from the beginning of the human race. There are specific combinations that God created and just mixed them up in certain specific patterns that created our individuality. Plus, He also added certain emotional traits that through the process of evolution and through the years have created unique qualities in each one of us. So our personality is the product of our genetic makeup, plus our emotional makeup modified by our interaction with others and our experiences in life. There are *basically six main energetic personalities* that evolved from our energetic makeup. These are further subdivided into 12 energetic personalities. Each "energetic personality" responds differently to external influences. That is why the effect of chemicals or medications is different from one person to another. We probably could enhance our Genetic Energy, but we cannot change it much. Our Genetic Energy is closely related to the kidney energy, the "battery" of the body, which are the adrenal glands. Any disruption of the Genetic Energy results in maldevelopment of the body, resulting in genetic problems, such as mongolism, cleft palate, deformities of the extremities, malrotation of the abdominal organs, congenital heart diseases, Siamese twins, diabetes, and congenital absence of organs (or extremities) or even the presence of extra appendages.

This Genetic or Original Energy controls the growth and development of the fetus and provides the internal clock for which the fetus is born, at almost exactly forty weeks from conception. So for God to propagate the human race (His angels), He has to create a mechanism, whereby the human person is conceived through the interchange of "sexual" energies between a man and a woman, and after that fixed period of growth and development, the fetus is born at a time that it will just be enough for the fetus to pass through the mother's pelvis. However, God also made some adjustments by softening up the cartilages of the mother's pelvis to allow for an extra "give" thereby allowing the fetus to be delivered. The mother's Original Energy (Yuan Qi), is the one that gives strength to the uterus to allow for contractions. This will ultimately thin the cervix and allow the uterus to expel the fetus without causing harm to the fetus or to the mother's uterus. All of these processes are predetermined and almost always occur at a predictable timetable. This is altered only when something happens to the mother, either doing some unnatural actions or taking in harmful substances like drugs, chemicals, alcohol, or cigarettes. This also results when the mother is exposed to harmful radiations, is inactive or lacking in exercise, which will alter or weaken her Genetic energy.

Spontaneous abortion is nature's way or the body's way of cleansing itself of poorly developed fetuses. When there is a developmental malfunction, which results in a deformed fetus, the internal mechanism of the mother's body (immune system) will recognize this and send extra energy to expel the fetus. This works as a function of purifying both the offspring and the human race. This is one of the inherent powers that God has instilled into our bodies. We don't have any control in this, but yet it is predictable. This is obviously affected by whatever happens to the mother during conception and during the period of pregnancy. The internal monitoring system constantly monitors the baby's development, and its needs, and protects it from harm. It is said that all the genetic impurities of the woman's body is passed into the fetus, especially the first pregnancy. It is, therefore, not unusual for the first pregnancy to be aborted since the woman's body recognizes any deficiencies or excesses in the fetus, and if the deficiencies or abnormalities are so great, then the energy of the Kidney Channel will stimulate the uterus to expel the fetus. This is probably aided by the inability of the fetus's Yuan Qi to defend itself from the mother's Yuan Qi. This is due to the absence of that inherent rhythm that normally exists between the mother's Yuan Qi and the fetus's Yuan Qi. So in a way, it performs a purification process, making way for better and purified fetuses to be born. Most of the time, the child born to a mother after she had a miscarriage are beautiful and smart children. This has resulted in the birth of children who are more beautiful, smarter, more athletic, and more innovative than the parents. This has resulted in an improved human race.

In pregnancy, the fetus is totally dependent on the mother for its Nutritional Energy or Rong Qi. It is, therefore, important that the mother should nourish herself well plus some in order to provide for the fetus. The mother should also be well hydrated to provide not only good nutrition, but also good circulation to bring the nutrition to the fetus.

There are, however, countless internal and external forces that affect the pregnancy. The internal forces are mainly emotional factors or stress and nutritional factors. Some of the external factors are alcohol, cigarettes, food and drinks, drugs, extreme temperatures and radiation. Harmful inhalants will also affect the pregnancy. The emotional factors are fear, worry, depression, anxiety, and sadness, even excessive happiness or pleasure. The emotional factors are called "internal devils" or "internal dragons" by the Chinese, while the external forces are called "external devils" or external dragons. The external dragons are hot temperature, cold temperature, humidity, wind or a combination of them. I added radiation as one of the external dragons.

CHAPTER V

Rong Qi

Nutritional Energy

"**R**ong Qi" is the nutrition that we take in to give us energy. This is also called **Nutritional Energy**. It is composed of food and drinks. Nutritional energy is the energy that powers us to be able to function, controlling both our involuntary functions as well as our voluntary functions. Rong Qi powers our autoimmune system, both our cellular immunity (white blood cells) and humoral immunity (immunoglobulins or antibodies). Humoral immunity involves the production of specific antibodies or substances that work against specific antigens or foreign bodies.

Our involuntary functions are our various bodily functions like breathing, heart contractions, digestion, hormone and enzymatic production, cellular growth and formation, immune and antibody production, excretory system (urinary and colonic), and others like sexual functions to some extent. It powers our healing processes. The heart is the most important organ involved with our involuntary function coupled with the lungs, constituting the circulation. The Kidney Channel or adrenal system is a major controller of this function, which includes the brain, the thyroid, the gonads (testicle and ovary) and pituitary gland. The thyroid gland is of course involved with energy processes and metabolism. The gastrointestinal tract, from the esophagus to the colon is a major part of this involuntary function, as well as the excretory system (kidneys). This timing system or the flow of Nutritional Energy (Rong Qi) is predetermined and fixed. However, since this is strongly affected or controlled by the sun (as directed by God), the timing then is arbitrary, highly dependent on the sunrise, probably different during the different seasons of the year.

Our voluntary functions are those controlled by our voluntary muscles, the muscles that we actively tell to contract. It is the part controlled mainly by the Liver Channel and Gallbladder Channel. It is mainly composed of the tendons, muscles, and joints. The Liver Channel also controls planning and decision-making, hence greatly influences the nervous system. Of course, the Kidney channel through the brain controls the voluntary functions of the body. These include the muscles of our face, the trunk, and the extremities, both upper and lower.

It is said that there is a flow of Nutritional energy (Rong Qi), which is from one organ or channel to another, comprised of two hours of maximum activity for that organ channel, and twelve hours, later, its minimum activity. This is guided by the sun through its ultraviolet and electromagnetic rays. It starts with sunrise before 7:00 a.m., which stimulates the stomach and spleen channels. This in turn stimulates the kidney channel, triggering the release of adrenaline (from the spinal cord) and cortisol (from the adrenal gland). These two hormones are the starters of the body, and it wakes us up. In adults, this is approximately eight hours after we go to sleep. Therefore, it is mandatory that we should be in bed between 10:00 p.m. and 11:00 p.m. This allows our body time to prepare for the liver to do its function by around 1:00 a.m. Bedtime should probably be 8 hours before sunrise. The Liver channel is involved mainly with detoxification (inactivating harmful substances that got into the body), synthesis of important body substances such as bile and storing carbohydrates in the form of triglycerides (fats). The Liver Channel is probably the main organ responsible for directing repair and healing of the body, as well as the synthesis and storage of certain elements, including carbohydrates, cholesterol, and vitamins. It is mediated by Vitamin D.

The Stomach Channel is supposed to function the most at 7:00 a.m., or shortly after sunrise. This is probably true for spring, but maybe different for summer and the other seasons.

Flow of Rong Qi or Nutritional Energy:

07:00 a.m.-09:00 a.m. Stomach
09:00 a.m.-11:00 a.m. Spleen (pancreas)
11:00 a.m.-01:00 p.m. Heart
01:00 p.m.-03:00 p.m. Small intestine
03:00 p.m.-05:00 p.m. Bladder
05:00 p.m.-07:00 p.m. Kidney (adrenals)
07:00 p.m.-09:00 p.m. Master of the Heart or Pericardium
                      (Heart Protector)
09:00 p.m.-11:00 p.m. Triple heater (chest, abdomen, and pelvis)
11:00 p.m.-01:00 a.m. Gallbladder
01:00 a.m.-03:00 a.m. Liver
03:00 a.m.-05:00 a.m. Lung
05:00 a.m.-07:00 a.m. Large intestine

This flow of Nutritional Energy (Rong Qi) is probably not the same at all times. This varies according to the season; therefore, it changes with the sunrise. The sun controls the biorhythm, the so-called "flow of Rong Qi", via the Controlling Energy.

The *Stomach Channel* is the first channel activated by the sunrise. It thus makes sense that in the olden days, breakfast had been considered as "the most important meal of the day." The stomach is most active between 7:00 a.m. and 9:00 a.m. (or with the sunrise). The stomach processes the food, and with the action of the digestive enzymes from the pancreas (Spleen Channel), the food is digested. The absorbed food is then acted upon by oxygen to release energy (process of oxidation). It is this energy formed, called Nutritional energy that is passed from organ to organ, or channel to channel circulating through the entire body within a twenty-four-hour period.

It has been my observation that people who skip breakfast are generally tired and lacking in energy. They also have the tendency of becoming overweight and tired most of the day with headache as a common malady. Pain problems, especially arthritic problems are also common in these people. When the food reaches the stomach, blood circulation is preferentially shifted into the stomach. After the food reaches the stomach, the pancreas starts releasing the digestive enzymes as well as insulin necessary for food digestion and metabolism. This is the realm of the *Spleen Channel (9am-11am)*. The Chinese probably mistook the pancreas as the spleen although it could mean both the pancreas and the spleen. Diabetics have spleen deficiency, hence, the spleen in acupuncture energetic could mean either or both the pancreas and spleen organs.

If a patient has severe coronary artery disease with insufficiency, then they are prone to develop chest pain after a heavy meal, due to the so-called "steal syndrome." This means that blood is preferentially shifted from the heart into the stomach—small intestine circulation in order to aid with digestion. Another way of looking at it is, next to the Spleen channel, the Heart channel is supposed to get the most of the Nutritional energy so that if there is a deficiency of this energy on top of an already weakened heart circulation, then myocardial infarction or heart attack can occur. This is probably one of the reasons that a lot of heart attacks or angina, occur in the morning, especially after a heavy meal. A combination of heart disease, increased adrenaline (especially in the morning) resulting in increased heart rate and a heavy meal can result in a heart attack. This I call as the Triad for heart attacks.

The *Heart Channel (11am-1pm)* is next to the Spleen Channel in receiving Nutritional energy. The Heart Channel needs a lot of energy to pump blood in order to aid the stomach and the small intestine in the digestive process. The Heart Channel and the heart organ are the main controllers of the circulation, body heating, and waste elimination. The heart pumps blood and heat to all parts of the body. The heart distributes nutrition and provides oxygen and water to the different parts of the body. After the organs and tissues burn the food in the cells (through the action of the supplied oxygen), then the waste materials are collected and brought to the kidneys (through the venous circulation) for disposal. The heart, therefore, is the main conductor for metabolism to occur by providing oxygen and nutrition to the tissues, help maintain a normal fixed body temperature through the circulation of blood (water) and finally, the heart helps our waste disposal system. This fixed body temperature is important because our organs, tissues, and the immune system are primed to function maximally at a fixed body temperature.

The heart pumps blood away from the heart to the different parts of the body to equalize the body temperature, while it also sucks blood from the body and back into the heart. This return circulation to the heart is carried out mainly by the contraction of the diaphragm with the aid of the intercostal muscles of the rib cage. This expands the lungs sucking the blood back to the heart. The contraction of the diaphragm creates a negative pressure in the chest causing the lungs to expand and suck air into the lungs while it also sucks blood from the periphery back into the lungs. The contraction of the muscles of the extremities, both upper and lower, will also squeeze the blood to go back to the heart and lungs. The return flow of blood from the periphery back into the lungs is aided by the presence of valves in the venous system preventing back flow of blood to the periphery. Understanding this anatomy and physiology will prevent a lot of medical problems, including blood clots, pelvic tumors, colon tumors, even anxiety and depression. Respiration causes the Lung energy to flow and help normalize body functions by also providing oxygen to all organs and tissues of the body.

After the Heart Channel, the *Small Intestine Channel* (1pm-3pm) gets the most of the "Rong Qi" in order to help it in its digestive and absorptive function. The Heart and Small Intestine channels give energy to the spleen and stomach to help it in its function. The Small Intestine channel helps the small intestine organ to perform its function of absorbing food and sending it to the liver organ for processing and detoxification. The Small Intestine channel, however, together with the Bladder channel is said to protect the outside of the body from harmful outside influences like cold wind invasion (common cold). It is said that it is the first channel that is attacked together with the bladder channel in viral infection or of common cold since these two channels protect the back.

The *Bladder Channel* (3pm-5pm) follows, emptying the bladder organ (organ function) as well as strengthening the entire back and protecting our brain (channel function). The Bladder channel is the first line of defense against cold wind invasion or so called "viral respiratory infections". The Bladder Channel surrounds the scalp, therefore, protects the brain. The bladder organ has to empty in preparation for the coming of more urine with its impurities. The Bladder channel runs along the back, therefore, one of its main functions is to strengthen the back and support all the other organs.

The Bladder Channel is followed by the *Kidney Channel* (or kidney organ) to get rid of impurities from our body through the kidneys, the ureter and finally to the bladder. The Kidney Channel functions best between (5pm and 7pm). The Kidney Channel allows the brain to function better through its channel function. The Kidney Channel also controls the thyroid gland, adrenals as well as the reproductive system. It controls the prostate, testicles, ovaries, and uterus. The Kidney channel controls the brain and is involved in our thinking processes. Somehow, it also controls the teeth, knees and bones, the ears (hearing), and the hair. Vitamin D is a very important mediator for the Kidney channel function. It is said that, "kidney vitality manifests in the moistness and strength of

head hair". Premature balding or graying represents a weakness in Jing."
Jing is the essence of life.

The next organ or channel that gets the major share of Nutritional energy is the *Master of the Heart Channel,* the "Protector of the Heart". It allows the heart organ to perform its function well, protects it from emotional stresses by allowing it to dissipate the stresses from the heart to the periphery, diverting excesses into the hands and giving it the energy to perform a multitude of tasks since the hands are extensions of our mind.

The next organ or channel that receives the Nutritional energy (Rong Qi) is the so-called *Triple Heater or Triple Warmer Channel (9pm-11pm).* This is composed of the body cavities, namely, the chest or the **upper heater**, the abdomen or **middle heater**, as well as the pelvic and retroperitoneal cavities or **lower heater**. The "upper heater" contains the two very important structures, the heart and lungs (and Master of the Heart), hence, it is mainly involved with tissue circulation, heating and oxygenation. The "middle heater" contains the stomach, spleen, liver, and gallbladder channels, which are involved with digestion. The third is the "lower heater", composed of the Bladder, Kidney, Small Intestine, Large Intestine channels, and organs involved in the elimination process. These organs receive a shower of energy to allow these organs to function in harmony with each other, especially with digestion and in waste elimination.

After the Triple Heater channel, the *Gallbladder Channel* (11pm-1am) receives its fair share of Nutritional energy. This not only allows the gallbladder to perform its function of releasing bile, but it also actively stores bile formed from the liver organ. Bile is responsible for fat absorption. The Gallbladder channel also strengthens the joints and tendons, healing them of whatever trauma it had endured during the day. The Gallbladder channel maximizes our ability to make plans. The Gallbladder channel is coupled with the liver, the liver being the producer of the bile that it stores.

The *Liver Channel* is one of the very important channels and it functions best between 1:00 am and 3:00 am. The liver organ is the largest organ in the body. The liver has many important functions such as synthesis of most essential proteins like albumin, carrier proteins, coagulation factors like prothrombin, many hormonal and growth factors, production of bile, bile acids and cholesterol, regulation of glucose, glycogen and lipid metabolism. It is also involved with detoxification of the body, storage of carbohydrates in the form of glycogen, as well as production of bile necessary for fat absorption.

The Liver channel is very important in the healing process. It is in charge of sleep as a channel. It is probably at night that healing occurs at its peak. It is, therefore, very important that we should be asleep long before the liver gets its Nutritional energy in order for the liver to perform its healing function. Thus, it is important that we are asleep before one o'clock in the morning for our body to be really rested. It is probably best to go to bed around 10:00 p.m. The nighttime is the time when the body grows, heals, and repairs itself. Sleeping during the day does not afford the same or equal benefits as night time sleeping.

In the olden days, we used to hunt for food during the day, do our chores of building, traveling, and gathering of food, playing, working, and farming. Daytime is the time when we raise animals for food as well as cultivate crops for food or harvest fruits and vegetables as well as go fishing. At night, we rest and procreate, this *God* accomplished by shutting down the daylight. It is at night that we regenerate our "batteries" (adrenal glands), heal our wounds and injury, as well as grow

The Liver channel also controls the feet and it helps the feet recover from its pounding during the day. That is the purpose that *God* gave these functions to the liver. Between 1:00 a.m. and 3:00 a.m., the liver functions the best in detoxifying the body as well as does its complex metabolic function. The Liver channel is also important in decision-making as well as in the proper functioning of the immune system.

In adulthood, we need approximately eight hours sleep in order to maintain good health. During illness, we need more sleep and rest so that we may need to take a nap also during the day. We should get up at approximately 6:00 a.m. or at around sunrise. The sun wakes us up and starts our "engine," ready to do our various jobs for the day. If people don't get up at sunrise or are asleep in the early morning, then they are prone to develop "heat" problems. Sleeping with the sun up means our body is already running in the "idling mode." As mentioned earlier, the sun probably stimulates the pituitary gland to release the Adrenocorticotrophic hormones (ACTH), which will start our "bodies' engine." This causes spurts or surges in the release of these hormones to start our body. If we do not get up with the sunrise, these surges are manifested by our waking up during sunrise and every thirty minutes to an hour until we will finally get up. It is not unusual, therefore, that we awaken every thirty minutes to an hour until we finally will get up. This overheats the body especially that they skip breakfast, as well as, missing on water intake. So these people have heat problems characterized by headaches and inflammatory conditions, including chronic diarrhea or any kind of painful conditions, like any form of arthritis. As mentioned earlier, they are always tired and lacking in **energy.**

People who miss breakfast are prone to develop obesity and chronic fatigue because they miss the energy that the stomach was supposed to provide to the rest of the organs of the body. This will also result in hypoglycemia or low blood sugar. The headache, therefore, could be the result of overheating of the brain, resulting in cerebral or brain congestion, hypoglycemia, and dehydration. This is worsened by the fact that they would mostly eat a big meal in the evening, between 7:00 and 9:00 p.m., the time of least activity of the Stomach channel. This results in poor digestion and assimilation, causing the food to stay in the abdomen; therefore, it is converted into abdominal and liver fat. This is worsened by the fact that a few hours later, the person goes to sleep and the body is in a **slow down mode**. This result is slowing of the metabolism. **It is,**

therefore, very common for people who go to bed late and get up late, missing breakfast and eating a big supper to be always tired, overweight, and have headache problems. They are generally obese and suffer from fatty liver or steatohepatitis with elevated liver enzymes. This illness is, therefore, self-induced.

The *Lung Channel* is next and works best between 3:00 a.m. and 5:00 a.m. It is not unusual, therefore, that people with asthma would generally have attacks early in the morning. The lung channel provides the body with the necessary oxygen to metabolize food, eliminate carbon dioxide, as well as help with maintaining normal body temperature. This temperature regulation is accomplished through the expiration of heat vapors through our breaths. The lungs also receive blood from the body for oxygenation and to release the carbon dioxide contained in the returned blood. The carbon dioxide (CO_2) is expired to the atmosphere where it is utilized by plants to form food. Animals eat the plants for their sustenance. Man eats the plants and animals to provide him energy for growth, repair, and proper body functioning. The plants in turn will release oxygen back to the atmosphere. This is a very important symbiosis between plants and man or animals. The interference of this important symbiosis through excessive cutting of trees and deforestations has contributed to many health problems that we have today.

As I mentioned earlier, the diaphragm is responsible for inspiration. Expiration is nothing more but the recoil of the thoracic (chest) cavity and the collapse of the lungs forcing air out of the lungs. Tight clothing (pants or underwear) and too much sitting with decreased activity has resulted in decreased lung excursions. The result is decreased lung expansion with the resulting decrease in venous blood return from the extremities to the lungs. So in people with small mouths of 4 cm. or less in width, and also with hypertrophied tonsils or enlarged tongue, when they become inactive and gain a lot of abdominal girth, then decreased diaphragmatic excursions will result. Enlarge tongues are seen in people with Spleen channel deficiency and are almost always tired and obese. The result is an out of shape diaphragmatic muscle with decreased contraction and frequent rests. This I call **diaphragmatic fatigue**. The so called "obstructive sleep apnea" is actually a case of diaphragmatic fatigue, and therefore the nomenclature should be changed to **Diaphragmatic Fatigue Syndrome** and not Obstructive Sleep Apnea. The apnea that results is due to the fatigue of the diaphragm, just trying to rest. The resulting gasping for breath is due to the accumulation of carbon dioxide causing the respiratory center of the brain to send a signal via the vagus nerve into the diaphragm. The result is the sudden violent contraction of the diaphragm followed by normal respirations with subsequent decreasing excursions of the diaphragm due to fatigue. Then the cycle is repeated. This is best treated then with heavy aerobic and abdominal exercises, frequent deep breathing exercises and the loss of abdominal girth. Continuous Positive Airway Pressure (CPAP) machines should be used only in conjunction with my recommendations. This is the reason that most mouth surgery to correct this problem has generally been unsuccessful.

The *Large Intestine Channel* works best between 5:00 a.m. and 7:00 a.m. It is, therefore, not unusual that most people move their bowels first thing in the morning. The Stomach channel also enhances the function of the Large Intestine channel. This explains the so-called **gastrocolic reflex**. The gastrocolic reflex means that after eating and the stomach is filled, then the large intestine is stimulated to move. It is not unusual then for a person to go and move their bowels after eating. This is an indication of good health, but moving our bowels usually occurs only in the morning. Going to the bathroom after each meal may mean an overactive Large Intestine channel, but again, it is part of the gastrocolic reflex. This may mean an unhealthy system or a very healthy system, depending on other symptoms. If this is associated with fatigue or swelling problems or bleeding problems or even indigestion, then there is something wrong, and this should be investigated. The person should be checked for diabetes, bleeding disorder, and stomach problems, including "gastroesophageal reflux disease" (GERD) or Diaphragmatic Fatigue

Syndrome. Regular aerobic exercises should be part of the treatment, especially between 5 pm and 7 pm.

Colon polyps, diverticulosis, enlarged prostate, uterine and ovarian tumors, excessive heavy menses (Pelvic Congestion Syndrome), gallbladder disease, pancreatic diseases and diaphragmatic fatigue syndrome result from the sins of modern society. Too much sitting coupled with tight clothing, too much inactivity and too much rich foods has created obesity problems and obstructions in the arterial, venous and lymphatic circulations. Hence the above diseases, and when coupled with decreased water intake and the consumption of too much soft drinks (soda or carbonated sugared drinks) has resulted in varicosities, blood clots, kidney stones and hemorrhoid problems.

CHAPTER VI

Wei Qi

Controlling Energy

The "**Controlling Energy**" or Wei Qi is the energy that we derive from the sun, which activates our Nutritional energy. The sun is the direct and indirect source of energy. Directly, its ultraviolet and other rays together with its electromagnetic radiation, causes the body to heat up and be charged electro statically. This Controlling energy (Wei Qi) protects the body from harm and external injury. This energy surrounds the body twenty-four hours a day, coursing along the so-called yang channels. It is said that it rotates around the body twenty-five times a day. This is probably the energy surrounding us, resulting from the stimulation of Nutritional energy (Rong Qi) to circulate it around our body. I think I have felt that energy circulate, and this is not related with our pulse or heartbeat, and is probably faster than ten per minute, depending on one's state of health. This energy apparently goes inside the body and concentrates in the liver at night where it intersects the so-called yin channels. This is the reason that the liver channel controls sleep. Anybody with liver problems would most likely suffer from sleep disturbances, either insomnia, frequent awakenings (especially between 1 am and 3 am), or excessive sleepiness.

As I mentioned before, the sea or ocean has basically three changes. The tide of the sea occurs slowly and represents the slow changes in a person's energy level. This change occurs over many hours. This is the same in the body, occurring very slowly. This is our **Energy Pool**.

The first waves in the sea are large and occurs many seconds apart. The energy equivalent in the body likewise moves rather fast, rotating around our body at a particular rate commensurate with our energy level based on the Nutritional energy. The faster it rotates the better. The more forceful it is, the better as well. This is the major active energy field that allows our organs to function. This guides the movement of our Nutritional energy (Rong Qi). It protects us from cold, heat, dampness, wind invasion, external force or trauma, as well as protects us from radiation. This I call the **Protective Energy** (Wei Qi).

The second set of waves in the sea is smaller, more superficial and faster. The equivalent waves in the body are barely perceptible and protects the body from microorganisms, such as bacteria, fungi, and viruses. They cover the body with an electrostatic barrier, zapping these microorganisms as they contact the body. They are dependent on the electrolyte status of the body, mainly sodium and chloride, the main components of sweat. This third Controlling energy (Wei Qi), I call **Electrostatic energy.** The three Controlling Energies (Wei Qi) are (1) Energy Pool (2) Protective Energy (3) Electrostatic Energy, are probably activated by the sun and mediated by Vitamin D, a steroid hormone.

The Indirect Wei Qi is that Protective energy that we derive from Nutritional energy (Rong Qi) through the energy absorbed by the plants from the sun. These we can call as "stored energy". Plants derive their energy from the soil (water and nutrients), carbon dioxide (exhaled by animals and man), and the sun. The animals (poultry, fish, mammals, and others) eat plants, which derived its energy from the sun and soil. The products from plants (fruits, vegetables) are passive storages of energy from the sun. When man eats plants, sea food and animals, this stored energy is converted into energy by the body. This converted energy is called **dynamic energy** which gives rise to the Nutritional energy. This is the energy that protects us from the constant invasion of microorganisms from the outside and gives energy to the body organs and tissues to do its function of healing and also in protecting the body against harmful radiation. **Dynamic energy refers to the Nutritional energy and Protective energy.**

This Protective energy could be the so-called **Astral Body**, which surrounds us. The astral body is an "energy field" created by the movement of energy around our body. There are probably two astral bodies; one covers the upper body or the **yang astral body** while the other one is the **yin astral body**, which covers the lower body. This yang astral body covers the circulation above the heart while the yin astral body covers the circulation below the heart. **The activities of these astral bodies determine the energetic strength of the individual.** It is probably only an inch to two inches in thickness from the surface of the skin. If there is blockage in the flow of energy, then this astral body will expand and becomes huge as there is stagnation of energy, causing pressure or pain. Headaches can produce significant expansion of the Yang Astral body commensurate to the amount of heat and pain which could extend to as much as 1-2 feet from the body.

People with good astral body circulation can be sensed as happy, energetic people who can exude energy and joy. They generally have pink color on their skin and are warm. Those that have depleted astral bodies can "suck" one's energy and could be cold and depressing with pale complexion. They generally have no ambition and very slow when they move. When there is obstruction of the circulation of energy (heat), then heat rises to the top or to the head and, therefore, results in headaches. To treat this, the head should be cooled down, the energy circulated (by removing obstructions), the temperature lowered down by rest, increased water intake, cooling of the body with cold water. Avoidance of further heating (no caffeine, sweets, or cigarette smoking), removal of constricting abdominal clothing plus movement of the lower extremities to circulate the heat to the legs and feet will likewise stop the headache.

Another important function of the sun, especially with its ultraviolet rays, is its ability to stimulate the skin to synthesize vitamin D. This is the only vitamin synthesized by the body through the sun's action. Vitamin D is synthesized as part of God's grand design. Vitamin D strengthens our musculoskeletal system: the bones, joints, tendons, and cartilages. It also strengthens the fascia (muscle envelope), creating insulation and promoting the flow of Wei Qi. As mentioned before, Vit. D is also involved with the immune system and probably with some enzymatic systems. Vitamin D, therefore, is very important for our existence, function, and defense. It is also said to be important for breast, colon, and prostate health, and it also promotes a healthy mood. In other words, it affects all the five phases in the five element acupuncture energetics.

CHAPTER VII

The Body's Energetic Flow

The body's energetic flow follows a definite pattern. This is predictable and actually helps in the treatment process. This energetic flow of both Nutritional energy (Rong Qi) and Controlling energy (Wei Qi) keeps the body healthy and protects it from injury, trauma, foreign organisms, outside energy forces (wind heat, coldness, humidity) or radiation. There are basically "six energy axes" and twelve "organs" where this energy flows. These six energy axes are grouped into three **principal channels**, and each channel has four organs attached to it with two energy axes. There are yin organs and yang organs, moving in a counterclockwise fashion in the diagram. Energetic blockage can result in early symptoms but with negative laboratory or diagnostic tests. As this blockage continues for a long time, then fixed lesions will result and would show in X-rays, laboratory tests and other diagnostic tests.

The *Six Energetic Axes* are:

- o   Tai Yang (Greater Yang)   : Organs are small intestine and bladder
- o   Shao Yin   : Organs are kidneys and heart
- o   Shao Yang   : Organs are triple heater and gallbladder

- Jue Yin : Organs are liver and master of the heart or heart protector
- Yang Ming : Organs are large intestine and stomach
- Tai Yin (Lesser Yin) : Organs are spleen and lung

Any manifestations of illnesses in a particular organ will ultimately lead to problems in the other organs, especially if the obstruction or the cause of the problem is not corrected. It is, therefore, imperative that early intervention is brought about by removing the cause of the problem and then protecting the other organs. This can be accomplished by employing the energetic massage, if acupuncture cannot be done, then supporting the body with the "healing triad". **This Healing Triad is: good nutrition, good circulation, and enough proper sleep.** This involves early big breakfast with light supper, preferably 3 meals per day, lots of water and exercise, as well as sleeping between 10 pm and 6 am. Of course, acupuncture is the best way to treat energetic obstructions.

The Triple Heater channel, also called Triple Warmer, is an acupuncture term for the three body cavities, namely, the thoracic cavity, the abdominal cavity, and the pelvic cavity. The master of the heart or heart protector is the acupuncture term used to describe the pericardium, the envelope of the heart. Probably, any manifestations of problems of the heart channel may indicate that the master of the heart channel has broken down. It is, therefore, imperative to protect the heart once manifestations of breakdown of the master of the heart are noted. Some of these manifestations are palpitations or chest pains. Heart problems may involve emotional problem like depression.

The movements of energy along the Principal Meridians are illustrated on the next page. The energy movement is counterclockwise in the diagram, following the direction of the arrow. The left aside are the Yang organs while the right side represents the Yin organs. The top organs are located on the upper extremities which are also Yang in relation to the lower extremities which are the bottom organs and are considered Yin organs.

Illustration of Principal Meridian System

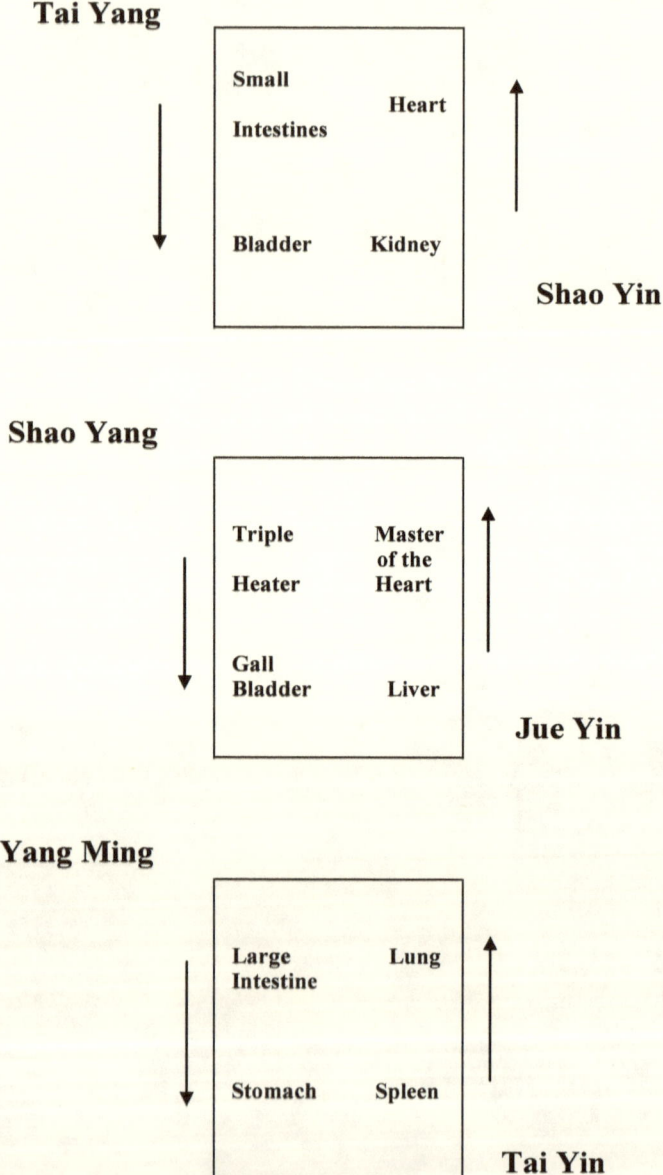

Fig. 1

CHAPTER VIII
Yin and Yang Concepts

Yin is the material part of the body while Yang is the energetic part. We can also say that Yang is the heating part of the body (energy) while Yin is the cooling part of the body. The Yin of the body is the blood, which carries the nutrition and oxygen, and the blood is mostly composed of water. God created life on earth with certain basic elements. They are carbon, oxygen, hydrogen, and nitrogen. Carbon, hydrogen, oxygen, and nitrogen are the basic constituents of amino acids, the building blocks of protein and of life. Carbon, hydrogen, and oxygen, meanwhile, are the major sources of energy, comprising the carbohydrates. Oxygen is the element necessary to burn carbohydrates and fats, and if necessary, proteins. This process of oxidation releases energy (quantified as calories), carbon dioxide (absorbed by plants), and water (neutralizes the heat produced). Protein is the basis of life together with carbohydrates and fats. However, in order to maintain life, carbohydrates should be burned in order to release energy to sustain body functions, therefore, of life itself. This does not occur without the presence of oxygen. *Oxygen, therefore, is the basis of energy production in our body. This energy release constitutes the yang or heating part of the body function. Yang involves heat production.* However, with the release of energy or heat, the body should be cooled down to maintain the constant normal body temperature of approximately 37°C or 98.6°F. It is important that a normal body temperature is maintained because the body tissues and organs, especially the immune system and the brain, are programmed to work best at that temperature level. This constant normal body temperature is accomplished by water absorbing the heat, then dissipating the heat to the outside through sweating, breathing, and urination. Bowel movements will likewise release some heat although not a major component. Bowel movement can become a compensatory mechanism or an emergency mode of eliminating excessive heat when the other basic mechanisms are shot down. Normal heat loss (sweating, breathing, and urination) can be impaired by the combination of excessive intake of heating items (caffeine, hot drinks, red meat, and sweets), excessive exposure to the sun, and inadequate intake of water. This I call a **heating triad**. This "heating triad" results in overheating, "then the body will blow a gasket," which results in illness. This is the typical "summer diarrhea," which I don't think is only caused by a virus. If a virus is cultured from the stool, they are just innocent bystanders that happened to penetrate the body through the dried and cracked mucous barrier secondary to dehydration. That is why, most of the time, the treatment is just intravenous fluids or just increasing water intake plus cooling the body down fast through rest and cooling blankets.

Water constitutes the yin, the very source of life, the main component of the circulatory system (blood). Water is the main component of the cooling system (yin). There is no life without water. Water is composed of hydrogen (yin part) and oxygen (yang part). Life is a balance between Yin and Yang. Nutrition is the source of Yang, the heating system of the body and Yin is the cooling system, mainly water. The Yang must, therefore, be balanced with the Yin to result in health or to promote healing by maintaining a constant body temperature through proper circulation. This fixed body temperature is essential for the proper functioning of the different organs and of the immune system, especially of the brain. The three basic needs of the brain that are essential to its function are water, glucose or sugar, and oxygen. Oxygen is more important than hydrogen;

therefore, two molecules of hydrogen are needed to combine with one molecule of oxygen in order to form water, the basis of life.

Ill health or disease, therefore, results when there is an imbalance of Yin versus Yang. Yang illnesses could either be an absolute Yang excess or a relative Yang excess. Absolute Yang excess is when there is an excess of heat (Yang), but the cooling system (Yin) is normal while relative Yang excess occurs when the Yang energy is normal or is slightly above normal, but the Yin energy is less than normal. Yin illnesses could also be either an absolute Yin deficiency or relative Yin deficiency. An absolute Yin deficiency occurs when Yin energy is low, but the Yang energy is normal, while a relative Yin deficiency occurs when the Yin energy isslightly below normal, but the Yang energy is slightly high. Most diseases are a result of Yang excess rather than Yin excess. Most Yang excesses are relative; they are the result of the combination of Yin deficiency or the deficiency of water, plus some excess heat. Most Yang excesses or heat problems are acute while chronic illnesses tend to be Yin deficiencies. Yang excesses are generally acute problems, sudden in onset. Examples are acute traumas, headaches, and diarrhea problems.

Relative Yang excesses tend to be chronic like arthritis or any chronic recurrent or persistent inflammation. The organ or tissues involved are generally warm but could be cold. The treatment for yang problems, therefore, is to draw heat from the body as well as cool the body down. Heat can be extracted by placing needles as in acupuncture or bleeding the patient with needle punctures. This includes incision and drainage as a form of treatment of abscesses. The body should be cooled down with cooling foods such as fish and vegetables, which, together with water, are very powerful coolants of the body. Yin excesses are generally manifested by coldness and edema. So any pain problem wherein the organ or tissue involved is cold with edema as a presenting sign, has a yin excess. They tend to be chronic. Yin excess results when there is a blockage in the energy flow in a weakened individual. An example is a chronic renal failure patient. They are generally cold, tired all the time, and are depressed. Chronic congestive heart failure is another example of a yin excess syndrome. Yin Excess is therefore characterized by too much water retention since the body does not have enough energy to move the water or enough body energy (either Nutritional or Controlling energies). Most excesses or deficiencies tend to be absolute in the acute stage but as it progresses to the chronic stage, then it becomes relative as deficiencies of other energies will follow.

Yang illnesses are manifestations of heat excesses, while Yin illnesses are manifestations of cold excesses. Examples of Yang excess illnesses are pain, headache, dermatitis, diarrhea problems like colitis or irritable bowel syndrome, arthritis, and acute trauma like sprains or any inflammatory condition. Most illnesses are heat problems. Osteoarthritis, on the other hand, is a relative Yang excess problem that is chronic, and the joint is generally cold. Examples of Yin illnesses are chronic renal failure, hypothyroidism, malnutrition, malignancy, chronic congestive heart failure, deconditioning or any chronic illnesses. Common cold is an acute yin illness or an acute wind invasion. The treatment for Yin deficiency syndrome is to increase nutritional intake including water and heat the body up with hot drinks and/or foods or drinks that are heating, as well as increase the circulation of blood through exercise. The treatment for a Yin problem, therefore, is to heat the body up. Red meat, sweets, ginger, and caffeine can heat up the body as well. Tea can likewise have a similar effect. Part of the treatment involves providing adequate circulation, therefore, enough water. We probably had worsened a lot of Yin deficiency by withholding water too much, such as in chronic renal failure.

To determine how much water is enough is usually a difficult question to answer, although it could be ascertained by monitoring weight, blood pressure, pulse rate, urinary consistency, skin turgor, and especially the tongue appearance. The tongue in patients with Yang excess (heat problems) is generally dry and red with a dark, yellowish, brownish coating. The patient generally feels warm or hot and dry with dry skin and even skin rashes. Those with Yin problems are generally cold and have no "energy", and are tired at all times. The tongue is pale, either dry or wet, small, and coated white. Yin excess disorders may mean that the patient has too much water in their system, but the circulation is impaired. They are generally cold and usually with cold symptoms like runny nose and congestion. Whereas in a Yin-deficient person, there could actually be lack of water with dryness and weakness, causing impaired circulation. One has to really distinguish the two, although it may be difficult to ascertain in certain situations.

Checking the pulse may also give an indication to the patient's problem. In patients with Yang (heat) problems, their pulses are generally "full and bounding" and maybe rapid. While in patients with Yin (cold) illnesses, their pulses are faint, generally slow or so called "empty pulses". By correlating the tongue and pulse findings as well as their appearance and their skin turgor, then we can determine if the patient has a heating (Yang) problem or a cooling (Yin) problem.

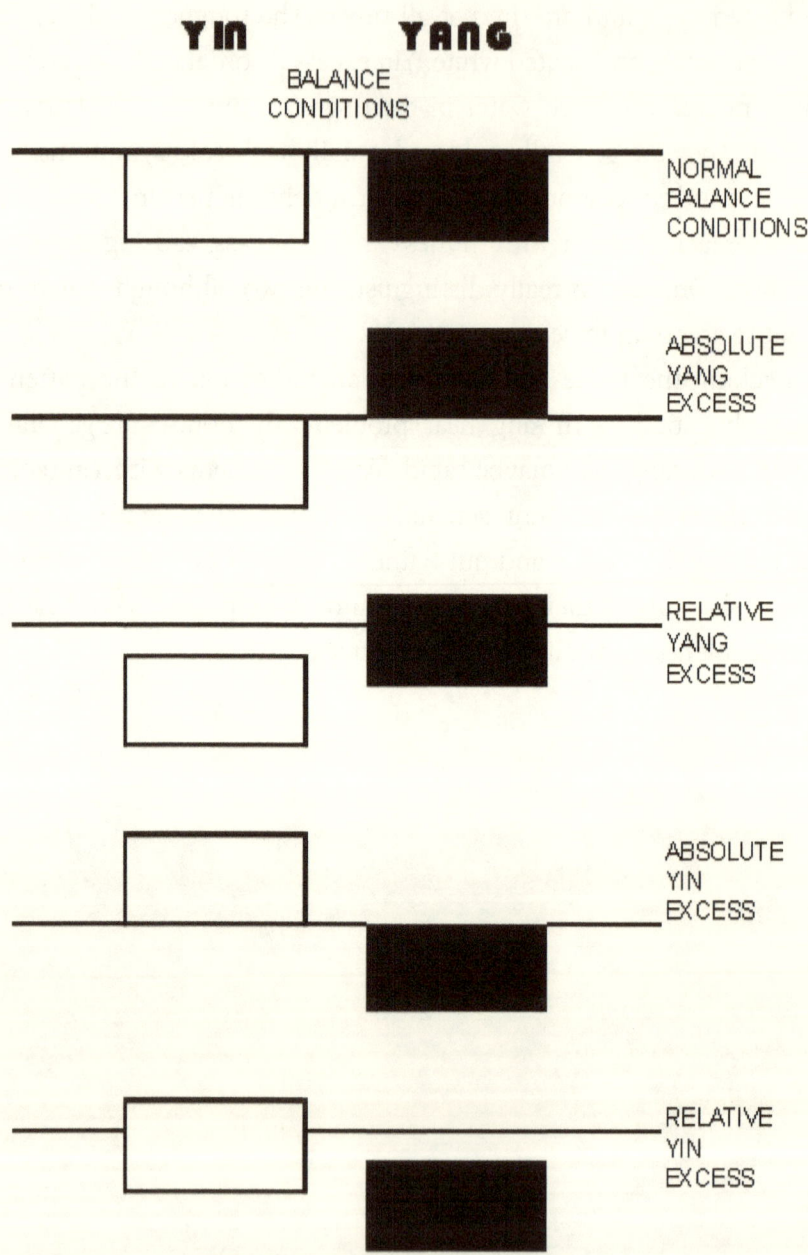

Fig. 2

CHAPTER IX
Yang Excess Syndrome

Yang Excess Syndrome means excess heat in the body. This results when the body is being attacked from the outside by any forces that somehow gained access to the inside of the body. These could be microorganisms, chemicals, wind, heat, food, radiation, or trauma. The body responds by mobilizing the body's defense mechanisms both humoral and cellular. This response increases the metabolism inside the body, in certain tissues or organs depending on the site of attack due to the body's immune system mounting a counterattack. This results in inflammation and or fever. There are certain chemical or cellular responses that occurs which results in the manifestation of the illness or malady. This does not necessarily have to be fully understood. *The body knows what is ailing it; and it also knows what to do to repair it.* For as long as the body has all the necessary means to attack the offending agent and repair the cell, tissue or organ damage, then all we need is to support the body to take care of itself. It is then essential that we provide the body with the proper support in the form of proper and adequate nutrition, adequate clean water and oxygen through exercise to improve circulation plus enough proper sleep. This does not mean that medications will not be necessary. Medications will support the body and its immune system in fighting the invading infection, but also allow the body's immune system to fight a decreased volume of infection.

We also need to rest the body or organ by avoiding its use to allow the healing process to occur. But at the same time, exercise should also be carried out to increase over all circulation, especially to the area involved. The earlier exercises are performed, the quicker the recovery will be.

The quicker we release any excess heat, the quicker will be the recovery also. Any acute disruption or interruption in the flow of energy or circulation will result in the accumulation of excess heat and blood in the area resulting in swelling. If we immediately decompress the area of this excess heat and blood and restore the flow of energy, then the return flow of blood and energy will be immediate. This will result in the body repairing the area quickly because the immune system is able to do its function. Thus in acute inflammatory conditions, it is important that the congestion of blood and heat be treated with decompression through bleeding of the area (or the use of acupuncture needles in sedation). This should be followed with the application of energetic massage but not ice or cold compresses. **If ice is utilized to shrink the swelling, especially if used for prolong periods, then chronic pain will result.** The object after the initial injury is to resume the flow of blood and energy. This is accomplished by the application of warm compresses for a few minutes followed by a short application of a cold compress (not ice). The warm compress will stimulate the flow of blood, but applying it for long periods will result in more swelling and congestion. It is important to apply a short cold compress (a minute or less) in order to shrink the swelling and force the circulation of blood and energy through the obstruction to help in the repair and healing process. This cold compress will also close the pores of the skin to prevent cold or wind invasion.

Energetic massage should be utilized as quickly as possible. Energetic massage is the application of light massage along the direction of the energy channel of the involved tissue. This is all you need and the application of ice is not necessary. Yang excess syndrome could also be treated by decreasing the intake of heating substances or foods like red meat, sugar (sweets), caffeine (and tea), chocolate, and even ginger. Yang Excess syndromes may manifest as feeling of heat, thirst, flushing, palpitation, headache, diarrhea or fever.

CHAPTER X

Yin Deficiency Syndrome

Yin Deficiency Syndrome means the lack of nutrients and or water. This usually results from chronic illnesses or malnutrition in poverty situation, or even in substance abuse cases. This is generally associated with kidney channel deficiency or adrenal insufficiency. These results in a weakened energy state, always feeling cold and tired with no appetite and depression is common. The resistance to infection is low, and the metabolism is slow. This is common in malnutrition, chronic congestive heart failure, hypothyroidism, and chronic renal insufficiency or kidney failure (dialysis patients). Other causes are chronic infections like tuberculosis, hepatitis, AIDS, glomerulonephritis as well as chronic parasitic infections like amebiasis. This occurs also in malignancy or cancers, like advance colon cancer, breast cancer, brain, liver, pancreatic cancers, especially lymphomas or blood related cancers. Their "energy" is very low, the Controlling energy (Wei Qi) and Nutritional energy (Rong Qi) are low, and the Genetic energy (Yuan Qi) is also depleted. As I said earlier, the treatment for Yin Deficiency syndrome is to increase the yin energy, and these energies are mainly supported by the kidney energy, liver energy, and the spleen energy in acupuncture (yin organs/channels). The other supporting energy channels are the Heart channel, Master of the Heart channel (heart protector), and the Lung channel. These energy channels can be supported with proper and adequate nutrition, enough circulation and adequate proper sleep.

The kidney energy controls the adrenal glands and thyroid glands, as well as the kidneys. These three organs are important in metabolism, energy production, and blood pressure maintenance. This is coupled with the heart, which is in charge of distributing this heat throughout the body thereby providing needed nutrition, oxygen, and water to the tissues. Blood pressure is thus maintained by the heart as well. The kidneys and heart supports each other in maintaining the blood pressure, maintaining body temperature as well as in waste disposal.

By increasing the yin energy, balance can occur, and healing will result. Another approach to a yin or "cold problem" is to heat the body. So for any cold or chronic problem, the energy should be increased by introducing heat or by increasing heat production. This could be accomplished by drinking hot drinks (drinks that increase heat production), eating sweets, red meats, or even drinking tea, ginger or coffee and especially through exercise.

CHAPTER XI

Heat Illnesses and Cold Illnesses

Yang Excess Syndrome and Yin Deficiency Syndrome are probably the two most common causes of illness afflicting the human race. Yang excess syndrome means excessive heat in the body while Yin deficiency syndrome means a deficiency in the cooling system or water but could also mean a deficiency in the function of an organ or of the body's nutritional status. In order to simplify things, it is probably easier to just classify illnesses into either *Excess Heat Illnesses* or *Excess Cold illnesses*; the other illnesses are just variations of these two illnesses.

Heat illnesses result when there is inflammation associated with an illness, or when there is trauma resulting in inflammation. Inflammation results when the body is mounting a reaction against an offending foreign body or there is trauma or injury to a tissue or organ. The body will then start the repair process by increasing the circulation to the area and sending immune cells to the area in order to repair it. Excess heat with swelling in the area of injury will therefore result. Heat could also be due to the breakdown in the flow of energy resulting in stagnation of blood in the area. Therefore, the area of injury generally gets cold at the onset, then will rapidly get warm and swell up. It is at this early stage that acupuncture could be very useful in decreasing the heat build up and resulting inflammation and prevent stagnation of blood so that the immune system can repair the damage quickly. The application of ice may work in the initial few minutes to prevent swelling but it will also prevent the reconnection of the broken energy flow. Therefore, the application of ice in trauma may actually predispose to chronic pain as there will not be any reconnection of the broken energy flow preventing proper healing. "Icing" should be avoided. Acupuncture should be used very early on after trauma or disease, not later. The longer the disease process stays, the more it firms up and become difficult to dislodge or clear.

Infection can also result in heat illnesses as the body mounts a massive response to the offending organisms. The signs of heat illnesses are fever, pain, swelling, redness, warmth, dry skin, absence of sweating, thirst, restlessness and finally, confusion may result. Confusion or coma is the end stage when the body's defense mechanisms and organs have failed. Heat illnesses can also result from too much exposure to the sun in the presence of water deficiency the presence of excess heating substances in the body like caffeine, sugar, red meat, cigarettes and even ginger. Other characteristics for these illnesses are pain, restlessness, sensitivity to touch or pressure, sensitivity to heat, maybe weight loss with poor appetite. Diarrhea could also be part of this syndrome and thirst is almost always present. Headache is a common presenting symptom. Excess heat illnesses are usually acute illnesses and the treatment is to cool the body down by the application of cold (not ice), avoidance of the heating elements and drinking lots of water. The heating elements are sun exposure, heating food or drinks and also excessive physical activity. Most heat excess illnesses are contributed by the lack of water; therefore, the intake of water is of paramount importance. Cooling the body down will allow the immune system to function and repair the tissue or organ damaged. The immune system works best only if there is not much heat in the tissue or the body, plus the ability of the circulatory system to deliver these immune cells and substances to the affected tissue or organ.

Excess cold illnesses on the other hand tend to result from chronic illness. It is generally a result of an acute illness burning out; therefore, it is the result of an organ or tissue being damaged from chronic inflammation resulting in decrease function of that organ or tissue. Examples of these illnesses are Chronic Congestive Heart Failure, Chronic Renal Failure, Fibromyalgia, Osteoarthritis, Chronic Fatigue Syndrome, Chronic Hepatitis, Cancer and many others. The hallmarks for these illnesses are tiredness with no "energy", feeling cold all the time, sensitivity to cold and could become pale and nutritionally deficient. They are generally sluggish, no appetite with weight loss and tend to swell up. This is a slow road to death.

CHAPTER XII

The Role of Emotions in our Health:

The Five Element Acupuncture Energetics

In "Five Element Acupuncture", every element has an emotion attached to it. There is also an important relationship between these elements. There are *five basic elements* in nature. These are the following with their corresponding seasons and emotions attached to them:

Element	Season	Emotion
1. Wood	Spring	Anxiety, irritability, anger
2. Fire	Summer	Joy, creative thinking, mania
3. Earth	Indian Summer	Introspection, worry, obsession
4. Metal	Fall	Sadness, depression, grief
5. Water	Winter	Fright, fear, paranoia

Wood generates fire, fire generates earth (ashes), earth generates metal, and metal generates water (liquid) when melted. This is the cycle of energy generation. There are two organs attached to each element.

In the "Wood Element", (corresponding to the spring season), the two organs or channels attached to it are the liver (yin) and gallbladder (yang).

In the "Fire Element" (corresponding to the summer season), there are four channels; two yang channels, and two yin channels. The yang channels are Triple Heater (triple warmer) and the Small Intestine channels. The Triple Heater channel is comprised of the three main body cavities, namely, the chest, the abdomen, and the pelvis. The two yin channels are the "Master of the Heart" (MH) or pericardium and the "Heart Channel". The pericardium envelops the heart; therefore, its main function is to protect the heart. Any afflictions of the heart may mean that the Master of the Heart broke down and is also involved.

In the "Earth Element" (corresponding to the Indian summer), the yang channel is the stomach and the yin channel is the Spleen channel.

In the "Metal Element" (corresponding to the fall season), the yang organ is the large intestine and the yin organ is the lung.

In the Water Element (corresponding to the winter season), the yang organ is the bladder and the yin organ is the kidney (and adrenals).

See the illustrations in the next page, which shows the Sheng Cycle (Cycle of Generation) and the Ke Cycle (Controlling Cycle). The illustrations will also show the different elements, the associated seasons, emotions, and colors. The different organs assigned to the different seasons or elements are also shown.

FIVE ELEMENT ACUPUNCTURE

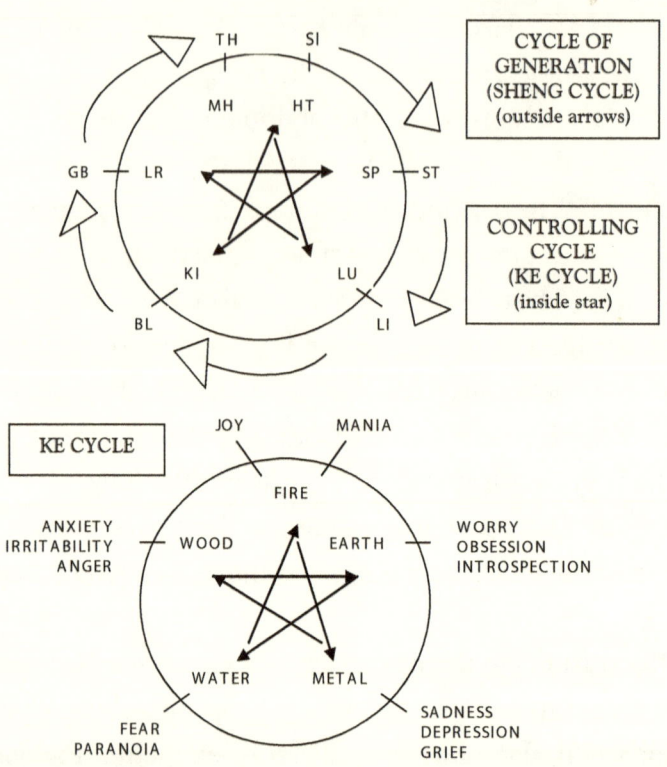

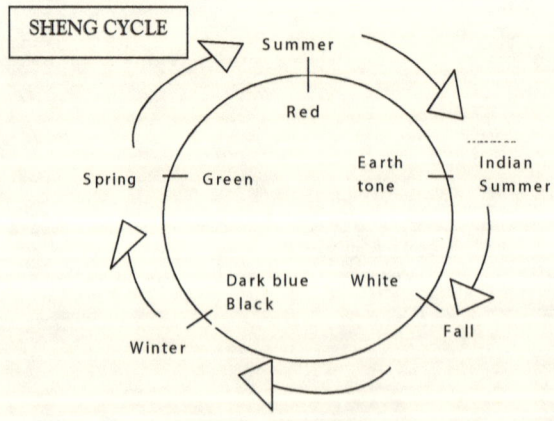

Fig. 3

As I said earlier, in the Five Element Acupuncture, there are five elements that represent the body's energetic movements. The elements that represent the body's energetic movements with their characteristics are:

Element	Season	Direction	Color	Emotion
Wood	Spring	East	Green	Anxiety, Anger
Fire	Summer	South	Red	Joy, Mania
Earth	Indian summer	Center	Yellow	Worry
Metal	Autumn	West	White	Sadness
Water	Winter	North	Black	Fear

In five element acupuncture, each element generates the next element. Everything starts with spring, the wood element representing the trees (green). The wood element generates the fire element. The fire element generates the earth element (ashes). The earth element generates the metal element (we get the metals from deep on earth). The metal element generates the water element.

Meanwhile, there is also a controlling relationship among these elements. This is represented by the "star" relationship. It is said that the water is the foundation of all the elements. This only reinforces the importance of water as the source or basis of life. The Kidney Channel is the yin organ of the water element. The kidney of the Kidney Channel includes the adrenal gland as well. I consider the adrenal gland as the "battery" of our body. It is said that the kidneys (adrenal glands) are the depositories of our "life essence" that determines our life span.

In the Controlling Cycle, the water element controls the fire element (puts out the fire). The fire element controls the metal element (melts it). The metal element controls the wood element (cuts the tree), the wood element controls the earth element (prevents erosion), and the earth element controls the water element (prevents flooding).

In review, there are two organs attached to each element except in the fire element where there are four "organs." In the water element, the yin organ is the kidney while the yang organ is the bladder. In the wood element, the yin organ is the liver, and the yang organ is the gallbladder. In the fire element, the organs are small intestine (yang) and heart (yin) as well as the triple heater (triple warmer), which is the yang organ and master of the heart (heart protector), which is the yin organ. The earth element has the spleen as the yin organ, and the stomach as the yang organ. The metal element has the lung as the yin organ, and the large intestine as the yang organ.

Each element could represent an individual's personality. We all fall to one of these elements with its characteristics, strengths and weaknesses. However, the personalities are subdivided based on figure 1, chapter VII.

In order to understand this relationship, you should study the diagram. If you understand this relationship, then you should be able to control your body. This is also important in performing the "energetic massage" to help cure an illness.

CHAPTER XIII

Energetic Personalities

Structural Biopsychotypes

Each element in the Five Element Acupuncture Energetics could represent an individuals' personality. We all fall under one of these elements with its characteristics, strengths and weaknesses. However, the personalities are divided based on Figure 1 on chapter VII. Dr. Joseph Helms calls them "Structural Biopsychotypes in his book, Acupuncture Energetics. According to Dr. Helms, the six Principal Structural Biopsychotypes with their subtypes are:

1. Tai Yang
    a. Tai Yang Fire
    b. Tai Yang Water
2. Shao Yin
    a. Shao Yin Water
    b. Shao Yin Fire
3. Tai Yin
    a. Tai Yin Earth
    b. Tai Yin Metal

4. Yang Ming
    a. Yang Ming Metal
    b. Yang Ming Earth
5. Jue Yin
    a. Jue Yin Wood
    b. Jue Yin Fire
6. Shao Yang
    a. Shao Yang Fire
    b. Shao Yang Wood

The characteristics of these Personalities according to Dr. Helms are:

Tai Yang structural Biopsychotype:

Level headed, intellectually lively, willful and decisive. They are leaders, balanced and effective in their actions. They are usually healthy and assume they can do whatever they set their mind to do. The Tai Yang person is generally muscular and sturdy and conducts himself with a frank and open demeanor. They generally have back problems generally precipitated by stress rather than by strain. They are sensitive, nervous and authoritarian person with too many responsibilities. They usually have sleep problems. **A sign of a depleted Tai Yang person is the inability to arrive at a decision or to sort out problems and options.** They could have abdominal pain with diarrhea and scanty urination, or other bladder problems.

Tai Yang Fire personality has excessive imposing presence with too strong a voice and too assured a demeanor.

Tai Yang Water person meanwhile, "is indecisive and excessively analytical. He knows what he wants but creates doubts and problems for himself in all dimensions, which prevent him from acting."

Shao Yin Structural Biopsychotype:

Because of the extreme polarity between Yin-Water and Yang-Fire represented in the Shao Yin energy axis, the structural biopsychotype is best presented in the Shao Yin energy axis. The structural biopsychotype is best presented initially into its polar expressions. In clinical situation, the pictures are usually polymorphous, containing aspects of both poles, but maintaining a predominance of one or the other expression.

Shao Yin Water patient usually presents with chronic or long standing knee pain or knee problems. Chronic knee problems are usually pathognomonic for Kidney energy deficiency. These patients generally have "diffuse low back pain that is improved with heat and movement and worsened with cold and damp weather. They have recurrent prostatitis, and a childhood history of recurrent tonsillitis. An affinity for salt is a manifestation of a Shao Yin Water constitution. They may have cold feet, recurrent cystitis, and darkness under the eyes. Men may have balding and graying hair with sensitivity to music and usually have tinnitus. They prefer black colors, have an affinity for salt and have inability to create a career. Their stamina is easily depleted by sex."

Shao Yin Fire patient usually have insomnia (due to excess heat in the head) and palpitation problems. Their insomnia could be accompanied by chest pain. They are usually sensitive to hot weather. They usually have cold feet and prone to have cystitis. They usually have high cheekbones, tall with flushed face and sweaty hands. Women are generally nervous and sexual with long well kept finger nails. They exude heat and likes red colors. Their tongue could have a red and raw tip, dry with a yellow coating at the base.

Tai Yin Structural Biopsychotype:

They are generally calm, neither happy nor sad and can appear introverted. They are clean and neat in appearance and fastidious regarding their personal environment. They are serene which could hide a brilliant intelligent person or a sluggish and lazy spirit. "He likes order, is prone to ruminating and obsessing over major and minor problems; his writing is very tidy, frequently small with generous underlining. He is sensitive to flavors and odors, and either strongly likes or dislikes caressing and being touched". Tai Yin women have strong maternal instincts. They like fresh air but fears drafts. They are a gourmand with affinity for sugar or sweets. Symptom of problems includes medial thigh heaviness, general heaviness of the calves, and edema of the lower extremities. They could also have fertility or menstrual problems, varicosities or lymphatic obstruction, flatulence or abdominal bloating, diarrhea and frequent urination. They could have anemia from excessive menses to complex blood dyscrasias and problems of glucose regulation.

Tai Yin Earth patients generally have problems with abdominal bloating, chronic diarrhea and recurrent vaginal yeast infections. Women could have painful and heavy periods with pre menstrual fatigue, irritability and bloating. They usually like sweets, women may have pelvic tumors; varicosities, anemia, cold feet but warm hands are also their presenting symptoms. They are generally rounded and fleshy in appearance with full red lips. They have short and square fingers, triangular finger nails, and chewed cuticles. They have prominent venous circulation and have a tendency towards ecchymoses and varicosities. They like yellow or earthly colors.

Tai Yin Metal patients usually have lung problems. They also have allergies and eczema by history (with chronic dry skin) and could suffer from chronic bronchitis, especially if they are smokers. They could have recurrent sore throats, and colds, chronic cough, easily gets short of breath, frequent sighing, allergic skin and respiratory problems.

They may have a strong family history of pulmonary problems. They also have bouts of alternating constipation or diarrhea. They could be well organized and methodical in the affairs of their lives. They are frequently plagued with depression, are generally tall and quite. They generally have narrow chest and shoulders, translucent or white skin and bad complexion. They could have long fingers, rectangular and slightly rounded with pink coloration. Their color affinity is ambiguous or white by default.

Yang Ming Structural Biopsychotype:

"A bon vivant person, knowledgeable about food and wine, who knows how to enjoy all the qualities of pleasure". They could have thumb arthritis, epicondylitis, shoulder and lateral neck pain, facial neuralgia, external genital pain or knee pain. They could also have anosmia problems or the loss of the sense of smell, rhinitis, and sinusitis. They could have dental problems, throat, esophageal, stomach, and intestinal disturbances as well as eating disorders. An anxiety-ruminating problem with falling asleep can also appear.

Yang Ming Earth persons can have elbow problems, specifically epicondylitis. They can have upper abdominal pain (left or right sided) especially after eating. They easily get an upset stomach, gets bloated easily and can become mildly depressed during the winter months. They can suffer from allergic rhinitis or some respiratory problems. They enjoy life and are full of vigor. They enjoy eating but have bowel problems. They usually have a round form, ruddy complexion but good skin. They could have a full and red tongue that is slightly eroded in the center but has no coating.

Yang Ming Metal person is "dry". They are cyclothymic or they have a bipolar mood with a greater tendency towards depression. They are usually thin and gray in appearance with bad breaths from chronic gingivitis and ill repaired teeth. Their tongue is always yellow and they have a "nervous stomach" with alternating diarrhea and constipation. They are generally tall and thin and appear depressed and lacking enthusiasm.

Jue Yin Structural Biopsychotype:

These people have chronic anxiety and emotional instability. They are inwardly nervous and chronically anguished. They find problems in every situation they are in. They continuously analyze themselves but cannot escape their problems. They have problems with migraines, palpitations and insomnia. They are restless, hold grudges and resentment and are capable of sudden anger. They are generally small and thin but not lacking in muscle. They have sweaty palms and cold extremities. They sweat easily and are sensitive to changes in the weather. They have affinities for sour or citrus foods like vinegar or grapefruit or for bitter chocolate or coffee. He can either feel exhilarated or exhausted from exposure to wind. Their hands and fingernails are well proportioned. You can usually see the "handkerchief sign" in women. They have foot problems, pain along the inside of the thigh and knee (medial aspect), and problems with the external genitalia. They can have headache or pain on the crown of the head, forearm and wrist pains such as tendinitis, muscular contraction or inflammation and carpal tunnel pains. Other common symptoms of problems in this type are cardiac symptoms of palpitations, chest pain and blood pressure problems. Cardiovascular work-up in these patients are usually negative. Digestive problems usually range from stomach pain to diarrhea, spastic discomfort and sensitivity to many foods. Migraines responsive or not to coffee are also common. They have insomnia and unstable sleep patterns. They could have liver problems like hepatitis, ductal problems as well as autonomic dysfunctions of many forms and patterns.

Jue Yin Wood person is inhibited, timid, hiding himself behind dark glasses and a wall that protects him. He never finds the words that exactly express his situation or feeling. They are anxious and inhibited with stiffness in their neck and shoulders with headache problems. Their headaches sometimes respond to coffee. The headaches are partly metabolic (Jue Yin deficient), partly biomechanical (rigid musculature), and partly endocrine (occurring frequently with periods). They are usually particular eaters with sensitive stomach. They become myopic at puberty with soft and ridged nails.

Jue Yin Fire person "is agitated, tense, locked into a tight and contracted framework from which it is difficult to externalize. He is irritated and angers easily. He can explode with violent and aggressive decisions and actions". They could have "debilitating chronic anxiety, disagreeable and unreliable moods, explosive anger, pounding heart, blood pressure sensitive to coffee, premature ejaculation, temporal and crown headaches, tight jaw, stiff muscles, and sweaty palms". They may be prone to addiction problems.

Shao Yang Structural Biopsychotype:

A **Shao Yang person** is a traveler. "His movement can be interior or exterior. It can be one of self-definition or of organizing and actualizing plans. He has an order that is unique to him, which may not be perceived by those around him. To disturb that individual order on the assumption that it is disorderly can cause grave injury to a relationship." Shao Yang persons are well built, often with well developed muscles, and are at risk for obesity after the fourth decade. They are prone to develop soft tissue problems on the forearm, scapula, ear, temple, occiput, upper and lateral thorax, intercostal muscles, waist, sacrum and hip, and lateral thigh and leg. Shao Yang symptoms are generally accompanied by the physical signs of myofascial spasm and trigger points. Shao Yang headaches can be temporal or occipital in location and can have radiation to the forehead and eye. They commonly presents with cervical and occipital problems concurrent with lumbosacral problems.

A **Shao Yang Fire person** is clear thinking and decisive, imaginative and productive (Yang phase). They are prone to muscle cramps. They could get anxious about completing projects by their deadlines. They are solid and talks quickly. They are directed and ambitious, and they make clear, fast and correct decisions. They are hard working, full of confidence and not afraid to make a move. They do not take measures to take care of their health but places confidence in nature and postpones making appointments for medical care. When they rest, they quickly regain their health and overcome any obstacles hindering them from living their intense life.

A **Shao Yang Wood person** (Yin phase) "is incapable of making a decision and circumvents issues and projects, to the frustration of those around him. He is capable of abrupt and untimely reactions and may show aggressive anger, but he can also harbor a bilious and enduring resentment. He is sensitive to ridicule and is inhibited when shamed. He is drawn to sour and citrus flavors", but he prefers green colors. He prefers morning for his activities, including sex and he prefers spring to the other seasons.

Importance of knowing one's energetic personality:

The knowledge of one's Energetic Personality or Biopsychotype allows the person to predict which reactions they may have to different situations, their weaknesses and illnesses they are prone to as well as be able to predict their reactions to certain drugs. A person's energetic personality will likewise determine how they react to things like trauma or medications. Different energetic personalities react to chemicals or medications differently, but each personality will probably react predictably to certain medications. It is best that we each know our energetic personality and that medication should be tested to each group to determine how a particular energetic personality will react to the medication. This will decrease drug reactions and complications. This may be difficult at times, but yet, an attempt should be made to classify our personalities.

CHAPTER XIV

Body, Mind, and Soul

The human being is composed of the **body, mind and soul**. This is how God created man, by giving us our body, which is the physical part of us. The mind resides in our brain, and this is the medium with which we think, express ourselves, create things, rationalize things and remember things. The soul is the invisible part of us that made us divine and ultimately is the part that goes back to God in the Heavens or to Lucifer in hell.

The **Body** is what we see and the medium with which we accomplish things and interact with other beings. It is the temporary part of us, the part that we have to physically nurture by eating, drinking and sleeping. It is the physical part that allows us to accomplish our mission on earth. It is the part that God has made as a temporary temple and residence of the soul. It is the part that gives us our individuality here on earth and separates us from each other. It is amazing that there are millions of people born but no one is exactly the same. It is the divine power that willed this. The body is the part that we shed when we die. Dying, therefore, is nothing more but the shedding of our temporary physical being. We eat, drink and sleep in order to hold on to our soul or spirit. Without this nourishment, then our spirit or soul will separate from us. There are of course many other ways with which the spirit will separate from our body. Anything harmful to the body will potentially cause the separation of the soul from the body such as physical trauma, chemical poisoning, infection, radiation, extreme temperatures and many others. This separation of the soul from the body means death

The **Mind** is the power that we wield, granted to us by God. It is the power to think and perform a multitude of things that God does not actively interfere with, except in certain special occasions. The mind is the intermediary between the body and the soul. It is not seen, its activity is not seen but it is perceived. The minds' power resides in its ability to synthesize words, concepts and emotions. We are able to interact with each other due to the power of our minds. This is the part of us that makes us similar to God. The power of the mind makes us think and do things that seem impossible. The power to talk, sing, hear, smell, taste and feel emanates from the mind or brain. It allows us to choose and make decisions. The brain is a repository of countless things including the capacity to learn and expand its knowledge, and the ability to train the body to do amazing things. The mind is the part of us that is capable to synthesize, invent and create things. The mind is the repository of our, experiences, knowledge and memories. The mind is the connection between the body and the soul, and ultimately with God.

The **Soul** is the divine part of us. It is the part of our being that is created by God and that will ultimately be united with God. It is the part of us that is being tested here on earth. The soul or spirit holds the key to our ultimate destination. It is also the part that can perform miraculous feats like healing, and the source of virtues like the power of love, pity, understanding, empathy and forgiveness and other emotions. The soul or spirit is the part of us that heals us, no matter what our illness is. It tells our body to physically heal wounds in the proper way and to heal our emotions when we are emotionally hurt.

The soul or spirit can be accessed either through prayers, meditation or hypnosis. Prayer is the active mental act of connecting ourselves with our Creator. Meditation is the active part of freeing our mind from any distractions, thereby allowing our soul to connect with our conscious mind and free our mind and body of any disruptions, including illness. Hypnosis on the other hand is the power of suggestion given by another person to us or by doing self hypnosis. When hypnosis is performed on us while we are in deep relaxation, then we can access our soul (subconscious) and give it the power to heal us or perform extraordinary things. The soul could perform healing through its effect on the immune system, or perhaps the immune system is part of the soul.

According to Richard Johnson, author of the book Body, Mind, Spirit, "sickness is not preordained or prearranged by any celestial power. While allowing sickness to exist on the material plane we call the earth, God does not choose particular people to be the unfortunate victims of it". I agree with Dr. Johnson. God gave us the free will to do almost anything we want, whether it is in coherence with or against the Rule of Nature. All the things we have invented and brought into this earth, God has allowed. Since He predicted these things to happen, He has endowed our bodies with tremendous protection and recuperative powers. He has also given the earth tremendous recuperative powers through the power of rain, sea waves, the ability of trees and plants to absorb carbon dioxide and provide us with clean air and oxygen. However, all through the years and the many harmful activities and creations we brought upon ourselves, has caused many illnesses that many times have caused death among us. Our inventions and lifestyle has resulted in accidents, poisoning, tumors and cancers, blood/bleeding problems, inflammations, immune disorders, asthma, allergies, organ dysfunctions like gall bladder, liver, stomach and pancreatic disorders and so many more. Many of these inventions involve food and drinks, chemicals, radiation and countless mechanical, electrical and nuclear inventions.

Dr. Johnson also mentioned Jesus Christ in his book. "Jesus used miracles to cure sickness and disease". If one will analyze the miracles Jesus Christ made, He used the power of energy, just as He felt His energy drained from Him as somebody touched His garment. Jesus used the power of energy to heal, and most of His miracles involved water, just like His first miracle of turning water into wine during a wedding reception, or healing the blind with His spit and soil. Healing therefore, involves energy and water, and blood is mainly water. The three main physical components of life are heat or energy, water and oxygen. Our inability to take care of our soul, and ultimately our immune system or healing powers, coupled with the abuse of our bodies has resulted in many illnesses and death.

We have to recognize that we are children of God, and therefore, have "powers" which are God given; we should use these powers accordingly. We should help each other and heal each other. But we have a responsibility to ourselves, to take care of our bodies and to respect it. We should avoid harming our bodies in the guise that we have the "right to do so". We have no right to destroy our bodies, but we have made our lives so challenging that it is very difficult to follow the Rules of Nature or the Commandments of Health. We likewise should take care of each other, for that is the main reason for our existence.

CHAPTER XV

Flash Signs and Symptoms

Flash signs and symptoms are signs or symptoms (one or more) that may indicate which particular organ or channel is diseased. These flash signs are important indicators of future problems. I have watched these and interviewed many patients, and I have come to the conclusion that these flash symptoms are accurate indicators of future illnesses.

Some of these important *flash signs and symptoms* are:

Kidney Channel problems or Adrenal Insufficiency:

The Kidney channel is the most common channel personality, and therefore, the most common presentation. The most common and important signs of Kidney Channel problems are knee pain, low back pain, and kidney problems like infections or stones. These are usually an indication that the person has indulged in early sexual activity. These may indicate future pelvic problems, diarrhea problems, dental problems, hearing problems, thyroid problems, bone and joint problems, and finally heart problems. Arthritis is also very common in later years. Balding is also an indication of kidney (adrenal) insufficiency.

Heart channel problems:

Emotional problems especially depression, bipolar symptoms, blood pressure problems, chest pain.

Small Intestine channel problems:

Indigestion or diarrhea problems, shoulder (back) or neck pain.

Bladder channel problems:

Back pain (hallmark), bladder infections, urinary frequency, eye problems.

Liver channel problems:

Foot problems, eye problems, and sleep problems, even anger problems.

Gallbladder channel problems:

Upper abdominal pain, muscle cramps, indigestion, headaches, indecision.

Spleen channel problems:

Tiredness, edema problems, varicose veins, heavy menses, indigestion, blood sugar problems, easy bruising.

Lung channel problems:

Asthma, shortness of breath, skin problems, allergy problems, sinus trouble, chronic cough.

Large Intestine channel problems:

Constipation or diarrhea, shoulder pain or problems, colic abdominal bloating or flatus, even "tennis elbow".

Stomach channel problems:

Heartburn or reflux problems, indigestion, eye problems.

When a person has a symptom, then other signs and symptoms should be looked for in that particular channel. This symptom should then be correlated with other symptoms or signs on that particular Primary Meridian (refer to chapter VII, fig. 1 illustration). One can then determine if the entire principal meridian is involved. The next step is to refer to the

Five Element Energetics to see which organ will be affected next, and to protect that organ (Refer to Chapter XII, Fig. 3 illustration).

Summary of steps to take to diagnose, treat and protect organs:

1. Identify the prominent sign or symptom.
2. Identify the channel involved.
3. Look for other signs and symptoms.
4. Identify the related organs or channel involved.
5. Identify the Principal Meridian involved.
6. Check if other organs or channels in that Principal Meridian are also involved. (Refer to Chapter VII, Fig. 1)
7. Check the elements involved according to the Five Element Acupuncture Energetics. (Refer to Chapter XII, Fig. 3)
8. Treat all the organs involved with Energetic Massage.
9. Protect also the next organ according to the Controlling cycle. (Refer to Chapter XII, Fig. 3)
10. Follow the Ten Commandments of Health. (Chapter XXI)

CHAPTER XVI

Taking Charge of One's Health: The Body Systems

It is possible to stay healthy by knowing how the body functions and then supporting those functions. There are eleven systems in the body, each system performing an integral part to the overall health and function of the body. Knowing how the body functions is essential in maintaining good health, protecting the body against illness and also in healing the body from illnesses. It is the responsibility of every person to know his body and to take care of his body. One should never surrender such responsibility to others, not even to their doctors. Physicians are there to help people heal from their illness, but it is the person's responsibility to keep their body healthy and help themselves heal.

The different body systems are:

1. Central Nervous System (The computer hard drive of the body)
2. Endocrine System (The messenger system in the body, controlling vital body functions and keeps homeostasis or balance in the body. Protector of the body)
3. Digestive System (The energy source of the body, which receives and processes food and liquid intake)
4. Respiratory System (Functions to provide oxygen in order to burn or oxidize food and eliminate carbon dioxide, the by-product of metabolism). Also helps with venous circulation.

5. Cardiovascular System (Responsible for the circulation of blood and nutrition, helps eliminate waste as well as control body temperature and blood pressure)
6. Excretory System (Mainly the kidneys, which disposes of waste materials through the urine)
7. Musculoskeletal System (The structural framework of the body, which allows us to move; gives form and mobility to the body)
8. Reproductive System (Responsible for reproduction and in maintaining the species).
9. Immune System (Cellular and humoral systems, protects the body from infection and outside foreign bodies, including eliminating cancer cells from the body).
10. Hematologic System (White blood cells, red blood cells, and platelets—responsible for carrying oxygen, carbon dioxide and other gases, fighting microorganisms, help with blood clotting and disposes foreign bodies).
11. Integumentary System (The skin which covers the body, responsible for our beauty).

These systems work in harmony with each other, producing balance to the body. These systems work harmoniously because of the balance of the yang system (heating system) and the yin system (cooling system), which results on a fixed body temperature of approximately 37°C or 98.6°F. At this temperature, the body organs will function maximally, especially the immune system. There is also a rhythm and balance between all these organ systems. The balance is accomplished by a rhythmic and uninterrupted flow of nutritional energy from one organ (or channel) to another. This is the movement of Nutritional Energy or Rong Qi, which starts when the stomach receives nutrition early in the morning. After the stomach energy, the spleen energy comes in (pancreas), which helps digest the food. After the Spleen channel, comes the Heart channel, which has to pump blood to the digestive system in order to help in the digestive process and in the transport of nutrition from the small intestines to the liver. The gallbladder pours bile into the digestive tract to help in the digestive process, especially in fat absorption. The small intestines are the next organ (or channel) that is activated to help in digestion and propel the digested food to the lower intestines while absorbing the nutrients.

The mixture of food materials being digested and the digestive juices poured in by the gallbladder and pancreas together with the acid formed by the stomach will digest the food and ultimately absorbed them in the small intestines. At this point, the organs of the chest (lungs and heart), the organs of the abdomen (stomach, pancreas, liver, gallbladder, small intestines), and the organs of the pelvic region (large intestines, kidneys, bladder) are simultaneously stimulated by the triple heater or triple warmer channel. This channel is stimulated to synchronously digest the food, detoxify it, transport it to the rest of the body, and remove waste materials. This is a different channel, which coordinates all these functions simultaneously. Disease or illness results when this harmonious and rhythmic coordination of function is disturbed or impeded.

Nervous System

The Nervous System is composed of the central nervous system (brain) and the peripheral nervous system, (the spinal cord, spinal nerves, and autonomic nervous system). The brain is the master organ, the main controller, the center of will, memories, emotions and thoughts and the control of our body functions; therefore it sits on top of our body and is encased in a hard protective envelop we call skull. It is covered with hair which physically protects it, act as protection against heat loss and also act as "antennae" to receive energy from the sun to enable it to function properly (electrostatic energy). These are the essential functions of the brain, which distinguishes us from other animals or from any of God's creations. This is the main similarity between God and us. He gave us that power to think, rationalize, communicate, formulate and create things and imagine things beyond what we can experience by our senses. We are able to invent and create things as well as solve problems. This is the greatest power that we have been given by God.

God probably gave us three basic powers. The **first** is the mental prowess, the **second** is the capacity to assimilate things in our body in order to nourish ourselves and to protect us from illness and the **third** power is the capacity to heal, both mentally, emotionally, and physically. We have tremendous powers to perceive things, analyze things, and finally create things based on these three mental capabilities. These gifts were given to us by our "Creator" from the beginning of time to support our existence here on earth.

Our central nervous system (CNS) functions as **receptors** via our senses, and as **processors** through our thoughts, telling our motor organs to do specific tasks. The brain protects us through the combined effort of our sensory, motor and autonomic functions. It allows us to feel pain and remove ourselves from the painful stimulus. It allows us to complete complex or even multiple tasks. It allows us to think, invent, or compose writings and music.

There are basically three functional parts of the nervous system:

- Motor Nervous System
- Sensory Nervous System
- Autonomic Nervous System

The **Motor Nervous System** generally is responsible for our willful actions. This controls our skeletal muscles, controlling our motor activities, including speech.

The **Sensory Nervous System** is responsible for our senses. We have basically five senses, namely, visual (sight), auditory (hearing), taste, smell, and touch. Our feelings or touch sensory apparatus detects temperature, either cold or heat and painful stimuli.

The **Autonomic Nervous System** is the "automatic" nervous system since it is not willfully controlled. The autonomic nervous system is composed of the sympathetic and parasympathetic systems. They basically control the heart and the vital organ systems, namely the digestive, cardiovascular, respiratory, genitourinary, including the body sphincters and sweating. The Autonomic Nervous System controls the heart rate, the caliber of the blood vessels, the size of the bronchial tubes, the function of the stomach and digestive organs, and the secretion of digestive juices. It also controls sweating, the sphincters of the anus and the sexual organs. It operates by way of sensors or "thermostats" located in the brain (brain stem) or the spinal cord. The Autonomic Nervous system operates through sensors and work via a balancing mechanism between the Sympathetic and Parasympathetic Nervous System, which works opposite each other, controlling the delicate balance of all these organs. The Autonomic Nervous system is also classified as part of the Peripheral Nervous system in some authors.

The **Exocrine System** is a system of glands and ducts which are under the control of the Autonomic Nervous System. The secretions they produce are poured out through a duct system (pipes). These are generally the digestive organs like the pancreas (digestive enzymes), liver and gallbladder (bile), sweat glands (and oil glands), prostate gland, and other minor glands like the skene glands in women's genitalia.

Endocrine System

The Endocrine System produces hormones that control vital body functions (the body messenger system). They pour their secretions directly into the blood stream where they travel into the target organ to control it. The pituitary gland is the master endocrine gland and acts as the thermostat for the functions of these endocrine glands. It acts as the sensor of certain specific functions, directing the endocrine glands either to increase or decrease hormone production. The endocrine glands modulate the activities of a particular system or organ in response to the body's needs. The pituitary gland is located in the brain.

The brain is the most energetic organ in the body. That's why it is surrounded by a lot of hair and protected by the skull. The pituitary gland is considered the master gland because it controls the functions of the rest of the endocrine glands. The different endocrine glands besides the pituitary gland are: the thyroid glands, parathyroid glands, the adrenal glands, the ovaries, the testes, the pancreas and the kidneys. The pituitary gland is controlled by the hypothalamus.

The thyroid gland produces **thyroid hormone** responsible for metabolism. The parathyroid gland secretes **parathyroid hormone** responsible for calcium metabolism, which is necessary for strong bones and teeth, as well as maintains integrity of the vascular system. The adrenal glands produce **cortisol**, the stress hormone and **adrenaline**, responsible for the fright and flight reflex. The adrenaline powers us for short bursts of energy waking us up and giving us energy to perform feats. The adrenals also form **aldosterone**, responsible for sodium or salt balance in the body. The sodium holds the water within the blood vessels in order to maintain the blood pressure. This works together with albumin, the protein that holds water within the blood vessels.

The other endocrine glands are pancreas, which produce **insulin and glucagon**, hormones necessary for glucose (sugar) metabolism; the kidneys, which produce **renin** in response to a low blood pressure in order to elevate it. Hence, the adrenal glands and the kidneys are responsible for blood pressure maintenance. Insulin will lower blood sugar while glucagon will increase blood sugar levels.

The pituitary gland operates by sensing the amount of circulating hormones from a particular endocrine gland. It will then order that target gland to produce adequate hormones according to the body's needs and balance. It is, therefore, very dependent on blood circulation (water), nutritional status of the body, as well as the temperature of the body.

The hormones produced by the pituitary gland with its target organs are:

- **Adrenocorticotrophic hormone** (ACTH) stimulates the adrenal cortex to form and release cortisol, a very important hormone for life preservation and functioning. The adrenal glands likewise produce adrenaline (adrenal medulla), which is also important in life preservation and energy production, mainly involved in the fright-flight response. The adrenals also produce aldosterone, responsible for sodium (salt) metabolism and maintenance of a normal blood pressure, and to some extent, it also produces estrogen and testosterone.
- **Thyroid Stimulating Hormone** (TSH) stimulates the thyroid gland to produce the thyroid hormones, which are important for metabolism or the burning of food for energy.
- **Follicle Stimulating hormone** (FSH) and **Luteinizing hormone** (LH) stimulates the production of hormones in the reproductive organs. It is also responsible for the production of eggs from the ovaries in women and sperms from the testes in men. The hormones released by the ovaries are estrogen and progesterone which are responsible for the menstrual cycle, while the testes release testosterone. Estrogen and testosterone are greatly involved with masculinity in men and feminity in women. Therefore, the imbalance between estrogen and testosterone is responsible for homosexuality and is not normal.
- **Growth hormone** promotes growth and development of the different organs of the body, and the body itself.
- **Antidiuretic hormone** (ADH) is responsible for controlling water balance by stimulating the kidneys to reabsorb water. It is therefore, important for blood pressure control and water balance.
- **Melatonin** is a hormone which mediates sleep and promotes a restful sleep pattern. It probably enhances liver function and is responsible for us going to sleep and staying asleep.

Homosexuality is an aberration of sexual hormonal production between estrogen and testosterone. It is not the fault of the person who has such a condition. There are a few factors that can cause homosexuality and should be approached with compassion and tolerance.

Digestive System (Gastrointestinal Tract)

The **Digestive Sy**stem starts from the mouth and ends in the anus. It is responsible for the ingestion of food and drinks, the mastication of food, digestion, temporary storage, and finally, the absorption of nutrients and excretion of by-products or waste products of digestion (feces). The main organs are the mouth, esophagus, stomach, small bowels or small intestines, and the large intestines or large bowels. The accessory organs are the liver, gallbladder and the pancreas. The main function of the digestive tract is to receive food, convert them into energy source, and pass it into the body mainly through the liver. It will also eliminate by-products of digestion or waste materials in the form of stool. The digestive system is the first channel activated after we wake up. It is, therefore, the job of the gastrointestinal tract (GI tract) to provide energy to the body in order to allow the body to function for the day. It is said that it functions best between 7:00 and 9:00 a.m., although it probably varies depending on the season. Eating a good breakfast (big and healthy) is important to give energy to the body. This also includes drinking enough fluids with breakfast and eating only to approximately 75 percent capacity of the stomach. How do we know that the stomach is not full? The absence of the feeling of fullness, churning of the stomach, and burping are signs that the stomach is not totally full and is able to churn and digest the food, releasing gas (burping). However, twelve hours later (7:00-9:00 p.m.), the stomach works the least so that we should eat less in the evening. We should not eat late (past 7:00 p.m.), just eat lightly and go to bed not earlier than three hours after supper.

At night, the stomach is already resting, and after we fall asleep, metabolism slows down, and besides, we are no longer active. This results in poor digestion, poor absorption, and underutilization of the food, in other words less metabolism. It is very common, therefore, for people who do not eat breakfast properly to eat a big late meal. If they are not very active, then they become obese and will have no "energy." If they do not drink enough water or they drink a lot of caffeine, then they are prone to develop pain problems (chronic inflammation), arthritis, or joint pain, especially headaches.

The liver is an accessory part of the digestive system. It is the storage organ for carbohydrates. It is the most important organ for storing blood and it regulates the volume of blood in the whole body. It also ensures the smooth flow of energy in the body. It contributes to our resistance against exterior pathogenic factors. "The liver is responsible for overall planning of the body's functions by ensuring the smooth flow and proper direction of energy (Qi").

The pancreas is responsible for producing the digestive enzymes necessary to digest carbohydrates, fats and proteins. It is responsible for producing the hormones insulin and glucagon necessary for glucose (sugar) metabolism.

Respiratory System

The Respiratory System mainly functions as the source of oxygen for the body. It is composed of the nasal passages, throat, trachea, bronchi, bronchioles and the lungs with its alveoli or air sacs. The lungs extract oxygen from the inhaled air and pass it into the body to oxidize or metabolize food to provide energy to the body. The respiratory system disposes of carbon dioxide, a by-product of metabolism. The lungs work closely with the heart. The heart and lungs are mainly responsible for heat production and heat distribution to normalize and distribute heat to the different parts of the body. The lungs also help in temperature regulation by expelling heat through the expired vapors.

The lungs, in conjunction with the heart, are the main keepers of life. Good lung function is, therefore, essential to life, for even the heart depends on the lungs to provide it with the necessary oxygen, an essential to life. Consequently, a good respiratory function is vital to the health and existence of the human body. Even a healthy pair of lungs is not enough to support good health if the person is unable to make good, adequate, and proper respirations. Shallow and irregular respirations can lead to disorders such as anxiety and depression, especially circulatory disorders such as varicosities of the legs or even blood clots. This occurs when coupled with dehydration and venous stasis from prolonged sitting or tight clothing, and/or smoking. Poor lung expansions and poor air exchange can also lead to tumors, edema problems, and lack of energy. The diaphragm controls the expansion of the lungs and the return of blood from the periphery of the body back to the heart and lungs. Poor diaphragmatic excursions result in lymphatic congestion which may result in colon polyps and cancer, ovarian and uterine tumors as well as prostatic enlargements and cancer.

Cardiovascular System

The Cardiovascular System (CVS) is mainly composed of the heart, arteries, and veins as well as the capillaries. The heart receives unoxygenated blood from the body and oxygenated blood from the lungs. The heart then pumps blood toward the lungs for oxygenation and away from the heart to the body to oxygenate the tissues and organs of the body. The CVS is a complex yet orderly distribution of pipes or blood vessels in the body, starting from large-caliber arteries to small-caliber arteries, and then to arterioles, which are very tiny vessels. There are also veins, which carry the blood back into the heart. There is also lymphatic circulation, which is mainly involved with the immune system.

The arterial circulation is maintained mainly by the heart, which pumps the blood away from itself. Therefore, the arterial circulation is highly dependent on the integrity of the heart muscle and its electrical system. The heart muscles are of course highly dependent on the oxygen that the lungs provide it. The arterial circulation carries oxygen, nutrients and water to the tissues and organs of the body.

The venous circulation is responsible for carrying the waste products of metabolism, mainly carbon dioxide (CO_2) and urea nitrogen. These waste materials are disposed of by the lungs (CO_2) and kidneys (especially urea nitrogen and others). The venous circulation or venous return, meanwhile, is controlled mainly by the action of the diaphragm or by the respiration. As we inhale, the diaphragm contracts, thereby creating a negative pressure in the thoracic cavity or the chest cavity. This negative pressure, coupled with the chest expansion due to contraction of the intercostal muscles and the suction effect created by the heart contraction, will cause the blood from the extremities to be sucked back into the heart. Since blood follows the law of gravity (all objects fall into the earth), God created a valve system in the large and medium veins to prevent blood from going back to the legs, or periphery (including the arms). The venous valves open up with the flow of blood from the extremity toward the heart and closes when the blood will rush back to the periphery during the end of inspiration. The integrity of this venous return is, therefore, highly dependent on the patency or free flow of blood from the extremities to the heart. Damage to these valves when blood clots occurs in deep vein thrombosis, prevents the valves from closing appropriately so that blood will back flow into the lower extremities causing leg edema. The heart also assists in this return of blood by its suction mechanism during heart contraction of the right side of the heart. The triad of tight abdominal clothing, prolonged sitting and dehydration will result in blood clots or deep vein thrombosis. This is especially true in obese people.

The lymphatic circulation is likewise dependent on the diaphragmatic excursions and also the patency of the flow of lymph from the tissues to the lymph nodes then to the thoracic duct and ultimately into the heart. The **thoracic duct** is the main duct (or pipe) that carries the lymph from the abdominal and pelvic cavity as well as from the lower extremity back into the heart, although this may not be present in everybody.

It is, therefore, important that we have adequate respiration (depth and frequency), patent veins, and lymphatic channels and a strong cardiac activity for the proper arterial, venous, and lymphatic circulation. Muscular contractions also aids in the movement of blood and lymph. This is very important not only in the distribution of oxygen and nutrients to the body, but also in the elimination of carbon dioxide and waste materials from the body. It is also important in maintaining a normal body temperature as well as in our immune function. So the three important functions of the heart and lungs are to: provide nutrition and oxygen to the body, eliminate waste materials from the body, and finally maintain a homeostatic normal body temperature. The heart also helps in maintaining a normal blood pressure. The blood pressure is dependent on three things; the heart rate, blood volume (dependent on water) and peripheral resistance. Peripheral resistance is dependent on the caliber, patency and flexibility of the blood vessels.

Excretory System
Kidney and Bladder Channels and organs

The **Excretory System** is mainly composed of the kidneys, ureter, and urinary bladder and urethra. The kidneys and bladder organs are coupled organs. The kidney channel in acupuncture energetics probably includes the adrenal glands, which sit on top of the kidneys. The adrenal glands are probably the "batteries" of the body. It controls the existence, function and life span of the person.

The kidneys are mainly responsible for filtering the blood and removing waste materials while filtering back important substances, especially water and proteins. It is, therefore, involved with water balance and protein balance (to prevent edema) as well as maintaining a normal blood pressure. It is also important in electrolyte balance, mainly sodium to increase the blood pressure and potassium which is important for muscle functioning or contraction. It is also important in hydrogen balance (control of acidity) and also in magnesium and chloride balance. These electrolytes are also important for heart muscle function. The kidneys are also very important in the function of the other organs, especially the muscles by maintaining a normal balance of electrolytes, mainly sodium, potassium, and magnesium. It helps maintain the acidity or alkalinity of the blood by controlling the balance of hydrogen, carbon dioxide, and chloride (pH of the blood). The kidneys are also involved in maintaining normal body temperature through its capacity to maintain water balance (urinary excretion causes heat loss). Therefore, it has a very important function of balancing the yin (cooling system) as well as the yang (heating system) of the body.

The bladder organ, in a sense, is only a reservoir of urine. Its function is of course dependent on the integrity of the kidneys as well as the influence of the organs around it, mainly the uterus, prostate, and urethra, and to some extent the small intestines (which put pressure on the bladder). The Bladder Channel protects and strengthens the back. It has its influence in all the inside organs of the body as well, being the main protector, but to a great extent, it also controls the function of the other internal organs, namely, the heart, lungs, liver, gallbladder, pancreas and spleen, stomach, kidneys, bladder, small intestines, and large intestines.

In Acupuncture Energetics, the **Kidney channel** includes the hypothalamus-pituitary glands, adrenal glands, the brain, the thyroid gland, reproductive organs (ovaries and testes), and as well as the ears, teeth, and the bones, especially the knees for walking. All these glands or organs are involved with life preservation, growth, procreation, and body functioning. These are the organs mainly responsible for metabolism, protecting us from stress, and helping us heal. The pituitary gland is the so-called "master gland" because it is our main thermostat, which monitors our vital organs via its control over the endocrine glands. The pituitary gland stimulates these endocrine glands to form the various hormones that mediate function of the various important organs of the body, including the reproductive organs.

Musculoskeletal System

The **Musculoskeletal System** gives shape to the body, supports the body, and makes the body move or perform tasks. It is governed by the Gallbladder Channel. The gallbladder organ is intimately connected with the liver channel. The liver channel, I think, is mainly responsible for apportioning nutrients to the muscles and tendons, healing and repairing damages to them. The muscles, together with the bones and tendons, are responsible for locomotion or movement. The muscles are composed of muscle fibers, which constantly slide against each other (actin fibers moving along the myosin fibers). The bones also move a lot around its joint connections. By natural law, anything that moves against something needs to be lubricated to make it slide better, to avoid too much friction, which causes breakdown of tissues, and thirdly, in order to cool down the tissues. Inadequate water consumption can, therefore, decrease the sliding of the tissues against each other causing a lot of friction. This results in tissue breakdown, and the inability to remove waste materials, which could then pile up forming arthritis. This also results in overheating which could lead to muscle spasm. Dehydration and overheating can result in headaches as well.

The **triad causing muscle spasm**, are: (1) overutilization of the muscle, (2) lack of nutrition (potassium, magnesium, sugar and or oxygen), and finally, (3) the lack of water. The lack of water is generally the final cause of muscle spasm due to decreased supply of nutrients and oxygen, accumulation of carbon dioxide, causing increased acidity of the muscle. This also results in the accumulation of lactic acid and urea nitrogen, resulting in further acidity. Overheating of the muscle also results.

The muscles and tendons are under the influence of the gallbladder channel while the bones and teeth are under the influence of the kidney channel. Vitamin D could be the bridge or mediator between the Kidney-Bladder Channels and the Liver-Gallbladder Channels.

Reproductive System

The **Reproductive System** is not active after birth. According to the Chinese, there is a "Rule of Seven" in females and a "Rule of Eight in males. The first seven years in females, eight years in males is a stage of rapid physical growth. The next seven years, eight years in males, is characterized by continued physical growth plus the growth of the sexual organs (seven to fourteen years in females, eight to sixteen years in males). The next seven years (fourteen to twenty-one years in females, sixteen to twenty-four years in males) is characterized by the maturation of the sexual organs). When a girl or a boy starts getting sexually active before their sexual organs are matured (ovaries at twenty-one years and testes at twenty-four years), then physical problems can occur early due to early consumption of the Jing energy (Original energy or Chromosomal energy).

Jing is said to be the **essence of life**. It is the energy that determines our life span and the degree of our overall health status. It apparently resides in the kidneys most likely the adrenals. We can liken this to rechargeable batteries. Rechargeable batteries have to be charged to the fullest before you can start utilizing it. This is because utilizing them before they are fully charged can cause a decrease in the life span of the battery. This is also true with the body. Having significant sexual activity at around fourteen to eighteen (true in both sexes) can cause a lot of predictable physical ailments. By sexual activity, it means ejaculations in men and orgasms in women, especially in women who get pregnant and deliver before twenty years old. Women who have a child at around sixteen years old are prone to develop knee pains (or arthritis problems), dental or teeth problems, back pain, hypothyroidism, pelvic problems, and even heart attacks or myocardial infarction (MI) and also stroke.

Women with early sexual activities or have babies early, frequently end up with a hysterectomy earlier in life. They are prone to severe arthritis, especially of the knees. They may develop Alzheimer's disease earlier. But another downside is the loss of sexual desire (and vaginal dryness in women). Men will also have similar problems of knee pain, back pain, prostate problems, hearing problems, heart attack, and even a stroke. Men will have erectile dysfunction or impotence (inability or poor penile erections) early on which could even affect them in their early 40's. It is, therefore, important to avoid sex before twenty one in girls and twenty four in boys. Short life is also a norm for these girls and boys who indulge in early sex. There is a rapid decline and early loss of sexual function with the concomitant development of major physical ailments. Does using medications like Viagra, Levittra or Cialis correct the problem? I am not sure, because forcing erection and ultimately ejaculation may actually deplete whatever remaining Jing energy is left. It is probably fine if sexual intercourse is only once a week to allow for the replenishment of the sexual energy. This needs further long-term study to see if it causes more physical ailments or if it actually decreases the life span of a man.

Having regular sex is in itself healthy. Being sexually active at the peak of youth (approximately twenty-one to thirty five years old in women, twenty-four to forty years old in men) will keep us healthy and young. By being sexually active, it means having sex about three to five times a week. Beyond this age, sexual activity should be curtailed to about one to three times a week. Sexual energy is like a well of water. When you draw water from a well, it will slowly fill up again with fresh water, slowly but surely. If you don't drain the well of water, then the water will become stale. Similarly, when a man ejaculates or a woman is stimulated and secretes vaginal lubrication and ultimately has an orgasm, then the "reservoir" is partially drained and then replenished with fresh energy and secretions. Having excessive sex daily or two times a day for weeks at a time causes rapid depletion, which may result to illness such as weight loss, kidney or bladder problems especially infections like cystitis, glomerulonephritis, kidney stones and loss of energy. Ringing of the ears (tinnitus) or dizzy spells may also result.

As we get older, the rapidity of replenishment decreases so that the frequency of sex should also be decreased. The absence of sexual activity is not good either, for that leads to a lot of illnesses related with aging and maybe, ultimately a shorter life span. Energy has to be released and replenished regularly. This helps keep the energy going, circulating, and refreshed in a natural rhythm.

Immune System

The **Immune System** is responsible for protecting the body against harmful invasions or microbial attacks. It protects the body from harmful organisms (bacteria, viruses and fungi). It also helps in the repair of the body after an injury, heals the body after an illness, and destroys carcinogenic materials in the body. It also inactivates or disposes of foreign bodies like molds, grasses, danders and many other foreign bodies.

The immune system is composed of the white blood cells and the immunoglobulins (proteins that fight infection and foreign bodies or helps heal the body). The immune system probably works best at night, most likely between 11:00 p.m. and 7:00 a.m. with its maximum activity between 1:00 a.m. and 3:00 p.m. This corresponds to the liver channel, which is most active between 1:00 a.m. and 3:00 a.m. Healing is maximum during sleep, especially at night when the rest of the organs are in a down regulated function. It is, therefore, very important that we are asleep at these times, especially when we are ill or stressed. Most people who are still awake by 1:00 a.m. will have difficulty going to sleep. People who sleep after 2:00 a.m. and who gets up after 9:00 a.m. are tired and frequently get headaches. This is due to three reasons, namely;

First, with sunrise, the sun's rays will stimulate the hypothalamus—pituitary axes to release Adrenocorticotrophic hormone

(ACTH) which stimulates the adrenal glands to ultimately release cortisol. Adrenaline is also released from the adrenal medulla (these are controlled by the Kidney Channel). The body and brain are, therefore, "idling" and running. This is the reason that most people will wake up every thirty to sixty minutes while in bed past sunrise. This is probably the reason that many people will dream during the early morning while in bed.

Second, since the person is still asleep at 7:00 a.m., then the stomach channel is deprived of food, which the stomach is suppose to have in order to provide nutrition to the person for proper functioning. The brain will not get the necessary carbohydrates either. The brain is very dependent on glucose for its function.

Third, since the person is asleep, they are unable to drink liquids, which are necessary to cool the body. Therefore, since the body and brain are "idling," then the patient heats up, needing more water to cool the body down.

Hematologic System

The **Hematologic System** is composed of three different kinds of blood cells. They are the white blood cells, red blood cells, and platelets. The white blood cells (leukocytes) are composed of the neutrophils (fights acute infection), lymphocytes and monocytes (fights chronic infection), basophils and eosinophils (fights parasites and foreign bodies). The red blood cells are responsible for carrying oxygen from the lungs to the tissues, then removing carbon dioxide from the tissues, and transporting them to the lungs for discharge. The platelets are responsible for plugging any leaks in the blood vessels, forming clots. Dehydration makes the platelets stickier and therefore predisposes the body to forming blood clots, resulting in heart attack, stroke, or gangrene of the extremities or the bowels due to blockage of the circulation. The blood cells are formed in the bone marrow; they are therefore, influenced by Vitamin D and the Kidney channel.

Integumentary System

The **Integumentary System** or skin surrounds the body. It functions as outside protection against foreign bodies especially microorganisms (bacteria, fungi, viruses) radiation and trauma; maintains the form and identity of the body as well as help maintain a fixed body temperature. It also aids in water balance as part of its function in maintaining body temperature and prevents water loss. The skin is also the vehicle wherein the Protective energy (Wei Qi) energy surrounds the body, flowing along the channels creating the so-called "astral body," which protects us from the outside invading forces such as microorganisms, radiation, and temperature extremes. The skin is the organ that synthesizes vitamin D through the action of the sunlight. Why is this so?

Vitamin D

Vitamin D is not actually a vitamin, but a steroid hormone since it could be synthesized by the body through the skin. It is the only vitamin synthesized by the body. Vitamin D has a major role in mineral metabolism. It is also absorbed through the guts from food. It is mainly circulating in the body bound to proteins formed in the liver (more than 80%). The vitamin D is finally matured in the kidneys with the help of the parathyroid hormone. So there is a close relationship between the liver and kidneys in the metabolism of vitamin D.

Vitamin D is important for calcium metabolism; hence, it is important in strengthening the bones and teeth and in maintaining the body's structure. It is primarily involved in maintaining the good health of our bones, tendons, cartilages, and muscles as well as nerves through its role in calcium metabolism. It is important for the immune system and is also needed by the heart muscle. It is one of the things that God used in order to support us by providing us with the sun. The ultraviolet rays of the sun stimulate our skin to synthesize vitamin D. The sun provides us with energy, food, and immunity. The sun wakes us up in the morning, helps us with our mood (preventing depression), and lights our way through the day to allow us to do our chores. The sun therefore controls life on earth and determines our life span as well. All these can only be done by a Higher Being—I call God, who other people call by other names, but is probably one and the same.

CHAPTER XVII
Maintenance of Normal Body Temperature

As I mentioned earlier, maintaining a normal body temperature is essential in order to allow the different organs and tissues to function at its best and to be able to synchronize its function with the other organs. In order to maintain a steady normal body temperature of 37°C or 98.6°F, the body has three basic mechanisms it uses to affect this. Heat loss from the body is mediated by water since water has a high coefficient of heat and is able to absorb a lot of heat per molecule. Mechanisms involved in temperature control:

The first one is *urination* or the loss of water through the kidneys. When there is excess heat, then the person will urinate more. This only works if the patient is well hydrated. If a person is already dehydrated, then the kidneys will decrease urine output by reabsorbing water. This is so in order to maintain the blood pressure, which is one of the main functions of the kidneys. Reabsorbing water may cause also the reabsorption of certain waste materials mainly blood urea nitrogen (BUN) and prevent the loss of heat from the body. This water reabsorption is mediated by the Antidiuretic Hormone (ADH), produced by the pituitary gland.

The second one is *sweating* through the skin. When the body is hot, then water absorbs the heat and expels the water or sweat outside through the skin pores, cooling the body down. However, if the person is dehydrated, then the skin pores will close, again in order to conserve water, which will cause the body heat to rise. Ultimately "heat stroke" results when the body is continually heated from the outside (like the sun or environment) or from the inside of the body, for example, by sugar or caffeine.

The third mechanism for temperature control is *breathing*. Expiration releases tiny molecules of heated water vapors. This helps cool down the lungs and the chest. Decreased respiration, therefore, will predispose the person to overheating problems like headache and pain problems. Decreased respiration will also decrease the flow of energy around the body and decreases oxygen supply to the brain while increasing carbon dioxide retention. This causes headaches, anxiety disorders, and circulatory disturbances, including Fibromyalgia and Chronic Fatigue Syndrome (CSF).

The *functions of the kidneys* are to:

- Maintain blood pressure
- Maintain body temperature
- Maintain electrolyte balance (mainly sodium, chloride, potassium, magnesium, calcium and phosphorus)
- Eliminate body waste materials (mainly blood urea nitrogen)
- Flush and cleanse the lower urinary tract, thereby preventing infection
- Maintain the acid-base balance through hydrogen or bicarbonate balance

The increased confusion that occurs in the elderly that has been traditionally blamed on urinary tract infections is basically caused by dehydration. Dehydration in the elderly causes a drop in the blood volume which results in a drop of the blood pressure. The elderly brain is atrophied plus there is a hardening and narrowing of their arteries to the brain. The low blood pressure and decreased brain circulation results in confusion. The dehydration also dries up the mucous lining of the urinary tract which allows bacteria in the urinary tract to penetrate the mucosa, hence, causing urinary tract infection. The initial treatment, therefore, is to hydrate the elderly and reserve antibiotic treatment only when the patient has symptoms of pain, bloody urination or has a fever.

CHAPTER XVIII
Hair Function

The body's hair has a very important function in the body. If we analyze the hair distribution in our body, one will notice that they are distributed mainly on the head as well as around the eyes, ears, mouth, and sexual organs. There are also some hairs around the anus, on the extremities, as well as the body. One will then wonder about the purpose of the hair as well as the relevance of its distribution. We can probably understand it better by knowing the effect of electrostatic energy on the hair. When we rub rubber on our hair, it causes the hair to stand up or the rubber to stick to the hair. The hair, therefore, acts as a conduit of energy, the so-called "static energy." It probably pulls outside energy, most likely energy from the sun or Wei Qi. The location of the hair also indicates an important function of these organs. The majority of our hair covers the head, because the head contains the brain, the central computer or controller of the body. The rest of the hair covers the sensory organs of the body, therefore, we see hair around the eyes (eyebrows and eyelashes), inside or around the ears (sideburns), inside the nose and mouth (beard and mustache). They are also located on the axilla, which is a very strong point of the Heart Channel, the beginning of the Heart Channel. They are also located inside the nostril to enhance the sense of smell. It also surrounds the main sexual organs (penis in men and labia in women), therefore, the thrusting action as the man has intercourse with a woman acts to increase the sensation as well as increases the circulation to the organs, thus helping in orgasm or ejaculation. The hair probably creates an electrostatic field which stimulates increase blood flow to the organs. The hair also surrounds the anus as well as in the fingers and toes. The fingers and the toes are where the "ting points" are located. Ting points are the entry points of energy in the body as the energy moves from one channel to another. The hairs probably act as "antennae" to receive electrostatic energy or electromagnetic energy from the sun or as a conduit of energy transfer or interaction. They enhance the function of the sensory organs as well as the orifices of the body. The hair also acts as conduits for heat transfer from the inside to the outside of the body as it directs sweat to the outside of the skin. Therefore, it helps in releasing excess heat from the inside of the body and or the organs to the outside.

CHAPTER XIX
Sexual Function/Activity

During the sexual act, the man thrusts his penis in and out of the woman's vagina, creating an electrostatic energy, which enhances the sensation and pleasure of the couple. This is coupled with the lubrication of the vagina, which probably results in the interchange of energy between the man and the woman until there is a build-up of energy around the penis and vagina, leading to orgasm in women and ejaculation in men. This buildup of energy causes increased circulation to the area. Ejaculation or orgasm does not occur if there is no buildup of electrostatic energy and increased circulation in the sexual organs, resulting from the thrusting motion of the penis in and out of the vagina. This electrostatic energy can also be manually reproduced by masturbation.

Ejaculation in men or orgasm in women occurs for a reason. After an orgasm or ejaculation, the woman or the man who had sex will be energetically drained. The man or woman will have to recharge before they can have the sexual act again. This process is similar to a "water well". To keep the water in a well fresh, one has to draw water from it. When the water level goes down, then water will replenish the well from its source. This keeps the water fresh. The "water well" almost never runs out of water unless under certain situations like drought. The laws of nature are the same. Therefore, ejaculation in men and orgasm in women refreshes the man and the woman. It ultimately keeps them relatively young although in the long run, we will lose our Yuan Qi with ejaculation and as we get older, our capacity to regenerate the Yuan Qi or original energy will end. This natural sexual act recharges the body and keeps the body youthful.

Sexual intercourse also harmonizes the energy flow between the man and the woman, contributing to the development of one being; both will become "tuned" to each other. This is to accomplish what God has said, that after marriage a man and a woman becomes one. They will then gain strength from each other as well as think or behave similarly, although they will not necessarily lose their identity and individuality. This creates love, harmony, and peace between the husband and the wife. It is not an accident that after lovemaking, there is more love between the husband and the wife, but not necessarily between a man and a woman that is outside of marriage. A man or woman who does not have this natural sexual interaction probably does not exchange much beneficial energies. There is an energetic difference between a man and a woman. We can liken it to the battery or magnet as having two opposite poles, a negative and a positive pole. The basic rule is similar poles repel each other while opposite poles attract. What is the reason then that gay men are attracted to each other as well as lesbians being attracted to each other? This is probably a result of an aberration in the energetic function of the man or woman during pregnancy, delivery or during the early development of the child. This is more apparent during the sexual growth and development of the sexual organs. This is most likely during the second and third phases of sexual development between the ages of eight to twenty one in girls and nine to twenty four in boys.

Homosexuality probably results from the damage to the Chromosomal energy (Yuan Qi) during conception or delivery. This could also be the result of immunization during early life, chemical exposure or the result of too much exposure to electromagnetic radiation from the outside like from microwaves, cell phones, radio waves, or television waves during intrauterine development, or during childhood. These waves generally don't affect the fetus or the child unless there is a lack of protection from the Nutritional energy of the mother or if the mother's immune function is abnormal. This results in the disruption of the Original energy based on the kidney channel.

The attraction and sexual encounter between similar sexes is, therefore, an aberration outside of the normal as ordained by God. The purpose of the opposite sexes is for procreation in order to perpetuate the human race. Sexual activities between two men and or two women are not natural; therefore, it does not result in the ordained consequences of the sexual act, which are pregnancy, recharging the body's energy, and maintaining a youthful appearance. Sex between same sexes is, therefore, a threat to the existence of mankind and their union is not a marriage. There must be factors that contribute to homosexuality. To follow my "triad," there has to be at least three causes. This could be a combination of the following causes:

Maternal Causes:
1. Genetic aberrations
2. Nutritional deficiencies
3. Poor maternal habits (lack of proper sleep, lack of exercise, poor eating habits, smoking, drugs, and alcohol abuse)

External Causes:
1. External radiation
2. Extreme temperature/humidity exposure
3. Trauma during pregnancy or labor

Environmental Insults:
1. Infections (bacteria, viruses, fungi)
2. Chemicals (drugs, medications, heavy metals)
3. Emotional trauma during the mothers' pregnancy or when the child is growing up (environment)

Any combination of the above factors can also result in the weakening of the Original energy or Genetic energy (Yuan Qi) of the fetus, resulting in aberrations or changes in the molecular or cellular structure of the fetus. This will result in imbalance between the maternal Genetic Energy and the fetal Genetic Energy (Yuan Qi) and, therefore, the fetal Yuan Qi is unable to hold on to its connection to the uterus (womb). As a result, the maternal Yuan Qi will expel the fetus, causing abortion or miscarriages. Similarly, when there is not enough maternal Nutritional energy (Rong Qi) to push the infant out during labor, then a prolonged and difficult labor ensues. This is very evident in late pregnancies (elderly women past forty two years) as well as pregnancies in multiparous women (multiple pregnancies uses up much Original energy or Genetic energy (Yuan Qi) and in women who had pregnancies early in their life (close to age fourteen). Early pregnancies (before twenty years) cause early use of the Original energy before the sexual organs are actually fully matured. This will ultimately decrease the Protective energy (Wei Qi) and protection against insult. The woman becomes sickly and ultimately has a short life span. This may predispose to the early development of Alzheimer's disease. This is also true for boys who indulge in early sexual activity, whether sexual intercourse or masturbation.

Women are unable to conceive in their later years due to the fact that their Original energy is depleted and their over-all energy (Wei Qi) is weak. Hence, they are unable to neither conceive nor carry a normal pregnancy. This is the reason that late pregnancies are generally miscarried or will result in deformed fetuses or they are unable to have a normal delivery. Caesarean section is common in late pregnancies.

CHAPTER XX
Water Balance

Sunlight, water, and oxygen are the keys to the existence of life on earth. Water is the medium with which metabolism occurs in the body. Water is the main component of the body's circulation or of blood, the main vehicle with which nutrition is carried to the different parts of the body. Blood also carries the oxygen to the tissues. Blood also carries all the waste materials (including CO_2) from the body to the skin, lungs, and kidneys for disposal.

Water constitutes *approximately* 60 percent of the body weight. Water constitutes the majority component of blood. *Blood has three main functions:*

1. To carry nutrition to the different parts of the body.
2. To remove by-products of metabolism or waste materials from the different parts (organs and tissues) of the body and dispose them to the outside through the kidneys, lungs, and skin.
3. To balance body temperature by cooling down overheated tissues and organs, to warm up cold tissues or organs and to lubricate tissues especially joints, muscles and tendons.

It is very important, therefore, to pay close attention to our hydration. The body knows what it needs to function and how it should function.

The body knows how to protect itself against diseases and heal after an ailment. Remember, in illness "*the body knows what is wrong with it and it knows how to fix itself.*" All we need to do is to give our body all the necessary materials for healing which are: *adequate nutrition, adequate circulation, and adequate sleep.*

Adequate nutrition involves providing the body adequate primary and secondary nutrition. The *primary nutrients are: proteins, fats and carbohydrates. The secondary nutrients are vitamins, minerals and phytonutrients.*

Proteins are responsible for the bulk of the body mass comprising the muscles, therefore, also responsible for locomotion.

Fats serve as padding and protection to the body, helps keep the body warm and also is a vehicle for the fat soluble vitamins, A, D, E and K.

Carbohydrates are the energy sources for the body, the main source of heat production and temperature maintenance..

Vitamins are substances needed to assist in body functions, acting as coenzymes in various enzymatic functions. They keep the organs healthy, especially the nerve tissues, blood cells, clotting, and as antioxidants.

Phytonutrients are from plants which are necessary for health maintenance, generally acting as antioxidants. They act to modulate the endocrine system by acting as precursors to endocrine hormones like estrogen and testosterone.

Adequate circulation involves a properly functioning cardiovascular system, excretory system, and respiratory system. A well hydrated body is a key to good body function. Dehydration is a major source of most of today's illnesses and maintaining good hydration is essential to good health.

Signs of Dehydration:

- Feeling of Thirst
- Dry tongue with yellowish-brownish coating in the acute stage, cracked tongue in chronic cases

- Dry skin with poor turgor
- Feeling hot but not sweating
- Decreased and concentrated urine
- Flushed and tired
- Problem concentrating
- Weight loss

CHAPTER XXI

The Ten Commandments of Health

To be healthy, there are certain things that we have to do. These things are predetermined from the beginning of time, from the time we were created. These are the necessary items needed for us to be able to accomplish our mission. The multiple causes of illnesses and diseases afflicting mankind is mainly our own doing. We cannot afford to disregard these illnesses, but again, this could be God's or nature's way of allowing the population to be controlled. The way we are abusing the earth and its resources will someday create a cataclysmic event that will wipe out many people and redraw the boundaries of nations. Again, in order to delay this inevitable event, we should try to go back to the basics as has been passed on to us. We should follow the commandments of health. We don't have any definite scroll of law passed on to us from God, although God gave us the "Ten Commandments." I can only surmise that maybe the original Commandments that God gave to Moses, which he broke after it was rejected by his people in Mt. Sinai, was probably the commandments for health promotion. God gave Moses a second set of Commandments, which this time involved stricter social and spiritual directions, which is probably more difficult to follow than the original set of "health commandments." Here is my attempt to promulgate what God might have written to us from many centuries ago, if not at the beginning of time. It wasn't written down because of the absence of paper and writing instruments then.

This so-called ten commandments of health is my own attempt at rediscovering what God may have wanted man and woman to do in order to safeguard our own health and ultimately our lives. This is not written any place else, and this could be right or wrong. But I believe that these things I mentioned here are what had been passed on to us from generations to generations but which are abandoned or forgotten by most people.

The Ten Commandments of Health

1. Thou shall eat nutritionally and properly.
2. Thou shall stay active (exercise).
3. Thou shall drink enough water (avoid unnatural drinks).
4. Thou shall sleep enough and at proper times.
5. Thou shall maintain proper hygiene.
6. Thou shall take care of your spiritual health through prayers and meditation.
7. Thou shall avoid overindulgence of food, sleep, and any unnatural things.
8. Thou shall not overindulge in early or too much sexual activity but indulge only in appropriate and regular sexual activity with the opposite sex.
9. Thou shall learn and practice the virtues of love, understanding, and forgiveness and never forget to help others.
10. Thou shall avoid the use of harmful, addicting substances. (drugs, alcohol and cigarettes).

To accomplish these commandments, it is important to follow the laws of nature as I mentioned in the energetic movements in the body, specifically the flow of Nutritional energy or Rong Qi.

This means that we should get up with sunrise, have a healthy big breakfast by 7:00 a.m., and have only a light supper by sundown (before

7:00 p.m.), not any earlier than three hours before bedtime. Our bedtime should be between 10:00 and 11:00 p.m. in order for us to get the eight hours sleep by waking time at sunrise. Exercise should be done preferably between five and seven in the evening to strengthen the kidney channel (adrenal glands). These things should prevent obesity, pain problems and emotional problems.

Drinking enough clean water will enhance body function, maintain a normal body temperature and help maintain a youthful look.

Adequate hygiene means regular body wash or shower to cleanse the skin of microbial agents and remove dirt which will allow for good energy flow. Brushing the teeth also removes harmful bacteria from the mouth and helps preserve teeth as well as conserve the immune function.

Prayers and meditation helps the body access our **healing powers** or immune system and strengthens our mind, body and soul. It also helps with our relationship with God our Creator and with man.

Overindulgence of any kind will result in illness as it damages the body and will also use up so much of our energies (Qi).

Too much sex will cause a depletion of the "Jing" or "Life Essence". Our **Life Essence** is what I call the "battery" of the body and it is considered to be the foundation of all structure and existence. "Jing" or **life essence** is the substance that activates and controls growth, development and reproduction. It resides in the adrenal glands. Early sex will also cause an early exhaustion of the "life essence" resulting in a lot of physical ailments and early death. **Life essence (Jing) and energy (Qi) are considered to be the structural foundation of the "spirit".**

Practicing the spiritual virtues will enhance the health of the mind, body and soul. It will strengthen the immune system and promotes a healthy relationship and interaction among us. This will allow us to accomplish our mission on earth.

Harmful substances, mainly cigarettes, alcohol and drugs by far are the biggest threats to mankind. Smoking related illnesses contributes to almost half of our healthcare expenditures in the United States.

CHAPTER XXII

Sins Against the Body and Nature

Our modern society has created and invented multiple "conveniences" or developed habits that has only created health problems for us. The many diseases and illnesses that have plagued us are the direct consequences of these, especially that we consider them as innate freedoms or rights to do these unhealthy habits. Until we deal with them, our illnesses will continue to haunt us and may contribute to the demise of the human race. Nature will continue to adapt to the things we do to it but for how long and when will we get the point of no return? Some of the ills of society contributing to our illnesses are:

1. The invention of addictive products like tobacco, alcohol, and drugs. Tobacco products have led to lung cancer, emphysema, heart attacks, strokes, peripheral vascular diseases, amputations, and pain problems (especially back pain), as well as chronic inflammatory diseases. Alcohol has caused dementia, liver cirrhosis, ulcer, accidents and cancer. These things, together with too much sexual revolution have caused illnesses due to exhaustion and damage to the liver. It has also caused damage to the pancreas, kidneys, brain, adrenals, thyroid, ovaries, prostate, large intestines and the stomach.

2. The invention of the motor vehicles including airplanes have made us sit more and become inactive. It has also increased the rate of fatal and serious accidents. It has caused people to be tired a lot. This has contributed to obesity, pelvic tumors, blood clots, swelling, stomach reflux, gall bladder, liver and pancreatic diseases, high blood pressure and many other illnesses.
3. The invention of chemicals, which we have added to our food and drinks as well as to a multitude of household and industrial uses have put a lot of strain to our organs and have poisoned them. They may have contributed to autism or mental retardation.
4. The invention of rich foods and drinks loaded with sugar and fat, even caffeine, especially soda (pop), which has contributed to diabetes, kidney stones, obesity, heart attacks and heart irregularities, as well as strokes.
5. Too much sex in television, movies and magazines has made people have early sex as well as promote too much sex. Too much prevalence of homosexuality and other aberrant sexual behaviors have caused a lot of emotional, mental and physical illness. It has also increased the rate of crimes, not only against women but also against children.
6. The invention of electricity, thermonuclear radiation and electromagnetic (and electronic) emitting equipments and appliances has bombarded our bodies with these transmissions, especially from satellites and transmission lines. Inactivity has decreased our resistance against radiations from television (transmissions and picture tubes), radios, cell phones, car and garage transmitters and others, including against the sun's harmful radiation.
7. Night jobs or graveyard shifts, have forced us to stay awake at night when the body is supposed to rest and recuperate. This has caused adrenal exhaustion and delayed healing and repair of the body through the interference of liver function.

8. The invention of tight clothing like jeans, has caused obstructions in the lymphatic, venous, and arterial circulations as well as compression of abdominal and pelvic organs. This has led to ovarian and uterine tumors, excessive uterine bleeding leading to anemia, prostatic enlargement and cancer, gastric reflux, diaphragmatic fatigue (obstructive sleep apnea), gallbladder and pancreatic disease, diverticulosis, colon polyps and colon cancer, and peripheral vascular diseases. Hypertension, arterial aneurysms, varicose veins, and blood clots, have resulted from this. Blood clots have resulted from the combination of dehydration, tight clothing and too much sitting. Miscarriages could also be attributed to tight clothing. Tight clothing in itself is not the problem; it is too much sitting, coupled with tight clothing and decreased activity.
9. The invention of television, radio telecommunication, and computers, has forced us to be inactive and be exposed to radiation. This has caused us to sit during the majority of our waking hours.
10. Deforestations and constructions of metropolis have removed trees, which are responsible for removing carbon dioxide from the atmosphere and releasing oxygen back to the atmosphere for man to inhale and utilize for proper metabolism. Excess garbage and waste materials have also caused problems. These have caused some oxygen deficiency and too much carbon dioxide retention.
11. The overutilization of carbon products (coal, oil, gas), which have caused alterations in the atmosphere, including changes in the earth's revolution and rotation around the sun. These carbon products (so called fossil fuels) were probably placed inside the earth to help maintain gravity and normal earth revolution and rotation. Burning these carbon products has changed the weight and density distribution of the earth, adversely affecting

its rotation. This has resulted in earthquakes, tornadoes and hurricanes. The resulting carbon dioxide emissions have overwhelmed our depleted trees and plants (forests) in absorbing the carbon dioxide (CO_2).

I am not saying that these things are necessarily evil, nor do I advocate that they be banned or eliminated. As long as we don't violate nature's *"Law of Deficiency and Excesses,"* then we should be all right. *The "Law of Deficiency and Excesses" simply states that we can neither undersupply our body with the essential elements, nor can we take in (or do things) excessive amounts of harmful things.* Less of certain things or overindulgence of something leads to illness. If we follow this simple rule, then our body should be able to adapt to things and repair itself quickly. This is of course contingent on us following the *Triad of Healing: good nutrition, good circulation, and enough sleep.* This should also be true in the way we use up carbon products so that we don't deplete the earths' mass.

It is unfortunate that society is used to twenty-four-hour service that we actually demand it. We keep hospitals, transportation system, emergency services (police, fire, and ambulance), convenience stores, entertainment places (theaters, bars, and sport centers), service stations, and government services open twenty-four hours a day. In a sense, it is necessary for jobs, but we just exchange it for illnesses.

All these sins we have committed against our bodies and nature could be defended against by knowing our energetic makeup, enhancing our energies through good nutrition, adequate circulation, and adequate proper sleep. We should also avoid things that will lower our energetic protective mechanisms.

CHAPTER XXIII

The Triad

Life and nature itself is controlled by what I call "Natures Triad." I believe this is so because God created backup systems to enable the body to overcome adversities or attacks without breaking down. "The Triad" is:

1. Nothing happens without any reason;
2. If something happens to the body, it is because we did something wrong (knowingly or unknowingly) or because of external factors;
3. For a disease or ailment to occur, *there has to be at least three factors causing it;* two contributing factors and a final precipitating factor.

The third in this triad is the key. If an ailment occurs, we should find the three factors causing the illness. Removing at least one of these factors causes some relief, and to cure the ailment, we should remove all three factors. There could be more than three causes of an illness, but only three is needed to cause the illness to manifest. Almost always, lack of water or dehydration is one of the contributing factors, if not the precipitating factor. Removing these causes of the illness allows the immune system to repair the body. This is the most important theory that I could impart to all, both the health practitioners and patients. Similarly, if we know the different factors that can cause an illness, then we could avoid getting the "triad." I call this triad, **Nature's Triad**, or "Dela Torre Triad".

The "triad" applies to a lot of things that occur in our body. If you go back to my texts in this book, a lot of things are in threes. Examples of the "triad" are:

- Essentials to Life: Nutrition, Water, and Oxygen
- Primary Nutrition: Proteins, Fats, and Carbohydrates
- Secondary Nutrition: Vitamins, Minerals, and Phytonutrients
- Essentials to Healing: Nutrition, Circulation, and Sleep
- Three Circulations in the Body: Arterial, Venous, and Lymphatic
- Three Main Functions of the Heart: Distributes energy or nutrition to the body, maintains adequate blood pressure and maintains temperature balance in the body.
- Functions of the Kidneys: cleanse the body of waste materials, help maintain normal body temperature, and help maintain the blood pressure.

The "Triad" was probably established by God to protect us. This He did by establishing back-up mechanisms to prevent us from getting sick or from dying as we go through life, especially since He knows that we are going to do "crazy" things.

These are just some of the "triads" in the human body. Knowledge of this triad helps in maintaining good health, and applying the "Nature's Triad" aids in removing illnesses or correcting them. One should, therefore, look for the triad at all times when solving a baffling condition. Illness almost always is a result of the "triad" and lack of water, or circulation is almost always present in all diseases. Proper hydration should always be maintained in illness, together with proper and adequate nutrition and sleep.

CHAPTER XXIV

Energetic Massage: Early Healing of Acute Medical Problems

The Controlling Energy, especially the Protective energy circulates around the body. This energy is the most superficial and can be felt or accessed easily. Acute medical problems can be improved or healed by superficial massages along these acupuncture energetic channels that are interrupted or blocked. This I call **Energetic Massage**. This can be accomplished by anybody as long as it is performed appropriately and immediately after the trauma or manifestations of an illness.

This energetic massage should be done along the energetic channel since doing it against the channel may cause no benefit, or may actually cause some harm. Acute trauma responds quickly to this maneuver, however, this does not replace regular acupuncture treatments. This should be done in the absence of a regular acupuncture treatment as soon as an illness manifests or soon after an acute trauma.

Energetic massage can be performed by anybody, including the person who has the problem. However, it works best when performed by another person who has a good energetic makeup or who has no significant problem. When this is done by another person who happens to have a chronic deficiency problem, then this will only drain the person giving the massage and may actually make that person ill.

The massage is done by running the hand along the channel, just barely touching the skin, almost like Reiki. Deep massage of the tissues will cause movement of blood or lymph in the deep tissues in a different direction or causes trauma to the underlying tissues or muscles. The massage maybe performed only for a few minutes and maybe repeated several times during the day. For chronic problems, the massage should be done four to six times per day for as long as the problem exists. It should be remembered that a person who has an illness of a deficiency type should not perform this massage to others since it may further deplete them making them sicker. Examples of deficiency illnesses are: any illness with weakness and/or coldness as a presenting symptom like hypothyroidism, chronic kidney disease, cancer, liver cirrhosis, blood problems like leukemia, "fibromyalgia" and many other illnesses of Yin deficiency.

Energetic massage can be done with or without any aids. However, I prefer using the massage with the aid of lotions, preferably either Traumeel cream (a homeopathic medication) or Voltaren gel.

In order to perform the energetic massage, please follow the direction of the arrows in the diagram in Figure 4 . . . Again the massage should be performed:

- as soon as possible after the injury or occurrence of symptoms
- along the energetic channel
- by applying lightly, using a cream preferably Traumeel cream or Voltaren gel. Other kinds can also be used.
- preferably by another person who has no chronic deficiency illness
- a few minutes four to six times per day
- should incorporate exercises with it
- following healthy habits, especially drinking lots of water
- stay warm and have adequate sleep

In cases of problems in the abdomen, like abdominal pain with or without colic, the umbilicus should be palpated or felt, and if it is cold, the simple placement of one's warm hand over the umbilicus may cause the pain and colic to disappear. Again this should be done as soon as the symptom is noted, preferably within minutes. For acute frontal headaches, the tip of the nose should be felt. If the tip of the nose is cold, then the midline of the forehead should be lightly massaged from the hairline (GV-24) to the tip of the nose. This should be done for a few minutes or until the headache subsides. Any acute spontaneous pain is a manifestation of an acute energetic blockage so that a simple "energetic massage" maybe enough to unblock this blockage. **No ice should be applied in acute trauma since this will interrupt the flow of energy and circulation.** A simple energetic massage may suffice to effect rapid healing.

Palpating or feeling the skin for areas of coldness is a very useful maneuver. Areas of coldness generally are areas of pain and means that there is blockage of energy flow to this area. These areas should be massaged along the energetic channels until it warms up. This should be regularly checked and re-massaged if the coldness returns. The area should be warmed with energetic massage plus the application of heat or massage creams.

Energetic massage may not work if:

1) Not done properly—applying the massage in the wrong direction, or applying hard pressure.
2) Done after the illness or trauma has taken its root (long after the trauma).
3) Patient's energy status is weak.
4) Patient's nutritional status is poor.
5) Patient is dehydrated.
6) Patient does not have enough rest or sleep.
7) Patient has a terminal condition.
8) The person administering the "energetic massage" is weak or ill.

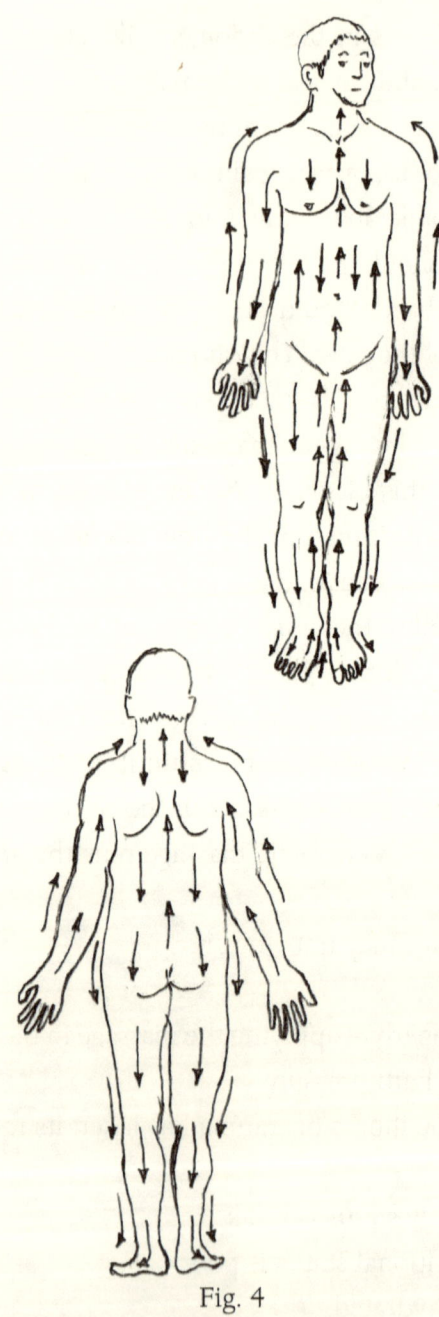

Fig. 4

Direction of Energetic Massage

(Follow the arrows which shows the direction of the flow of energy)

CHAPTER XXV
The Conclusion

Life was created by a Higher Being who found a reason to create man. I am a believer that our **Creator** did not create us without any reason, nor did we just accidentally pop out in this world. Yes, we probably descended from the apes, not by biological evolution, but by evolution of creation. God probably created the apes first, not wanting to create a being like Him initially because, according to the Bible, God's first creation was Lucifer (Satan), who was created a "perfect" angel that he thought he could become a god and does not have to serve God. So God banished him to hell. After God created the **Archangels**, St. Michael, St. Gabriel and St. Raphael, God probably thought it best to test his angels first before bringing them into heaven. So He decided to create His next angels and brought them to earth in order to be tested first if they are worthy to be brought to heaven. So when He created man, He sent us to earth, but not after He created all the necessary support systems that we needed. Yes, He did not wish to give us heaven outright, unlike, what He gave the original angels; we had to earn our "wings." Thus, He created everything around us in six days, all in order to provide us with all the necessary provisions for us to survive on this earth. Hence, almost everything we see with few exceptions (freak of nature) serves us in three ways. They are either for food or nutrition, for medicinal purposes, or for beauty (as food for the soul). God created everything and made the sun as the center of our universe, the source of energy and life.

The sun is the source of light, the source of energy and ultimately, our source of food. The sun is the cause of the day and night as well as the cause of the seasons. The sun is responsible for the plants and trees to bear fruits; the grass, trees, and plants are our sources of food. The sun heats up the earth for three reasons:

- To keep us warm
- To heat the earth's crust, creating electromagnetic forces responsible for the earth's gravitational force, this interacts with the sun
- Heats the land and the oceans in order to rotate the earth along its axis and revolve around the sun.

It is not an accident that life exists and that things around us behave at a fixed pattern. It is because our bodies are totally dependent on nature and how things behave around us. It is, therefore, very important that we tap into this rhythm of life in order to be healthy. Going against this rhythm of nature causes significant problems for us. It is not an accident that sunrise occurs in the morning, or that we have to sleep at night. It is not an accident either that we get hungry at certain times, or that we have sexual urges relative to the opposite sex (same sex attraction is an aberration). Our physiologic functions (eating, sleeping, urination, bowel movement, sexual abilities, breathing) are not by accident nor are trivial. They are the reason we are alive and the reason for good health. It is not an accident either that our parents contributed one set of chromosomes each (either X or Y chromosomes), and out of these cells (ovum or egg in females and sperm in males), a fetus develops and is delivered at approximately nine months or forty weeks. That is because that is the size of the fetus that can safely be delivered by the mother through the vagina. Then we grow to adulthood, learning vast knowledge peaking at middle age, and then we start to deteriorate. These are all predetermined by our "Maker." Why is this so? Perhaps because we are given a mission on earth, and we have only a certain amount of time to accomplish this.

God carried out all these by establishing certain rules and principles of nature. I can only surmise that the purpose of our existence is nothing more but to help others attain the Kingdom of God. To help others and help others be saved is probably our noble test and mission. That is probably why people who are concerned with others and do help others, are more satisfied, healthier, and happier compared to people who are only thinking of themselves and are therefore, selfish. That is not our nature and not the way we were made. We are not meant to only take care of ourselves, but mainly others. People who are self-centered tend to be depressed and dissatisfied, no matter what. People who are outgoing and are very willing to share things with others or who help others more, tend to be happier and more satisfied. There are of course exceptions to this rule, especially if they do not follow the rule to the letter.

Life and health, therefore, means following our role on earth and following the **rules of nature** in order to stay healthy and, therefore, be able to accomplish our mission on earth as mandated by our God or "Creator." Destroying our body or other beings is contrary to our purpose and mission. My role here is to try to point out to you and remind everybody of our role and mission on earth and how to accomplish it. Only by following the "guides" given to us as handed down from generation to generation, can we attain the greatest accomplishment of all, and that is to finally join our Creator in paradise as He originally envisioned for us. One of the great gifts that God gave us is the knowledge of Acupuncture Energetics, which is nothing more but **nature healing**.

Another purpose of this book is to help in preserving life and humanity. The ever expansion of the human population and the lack of personal responsibility in taking care of our health and of nature has threatened human existence and the world as we know of. Destroying life and resources out of hate, jealousy, and retaliation is against God's will and mandate. The ever-expanding monetary deficits among individuals, corporations, and governments have threatened our society. Greed, corruption, and overindulgence have corrupted us, causing moral degeneration. Inactivity, too much television, computers and games, and too much self-indulgence or gratification is ruining us. No civilization in history has lasted perpetually, ranging from the Greeks, the Ottomans, the Persians, the Romans, the Spanish, and English empires have all fallen down from the top. Is the American "empire" or influence crumbling down? It will eventually, but let us hope that we will have the strength, the courage, and the determination to work hard at it and postpone the inevitable. But this ultimately need to start from **"the man on the mirror"** (or woman). Only by taking care of our health, taking care of others, and caring for each other can we improve the health of our society and decrease the budget deficit. This will improve the well-being of not only the American people, but of all the people in the world.

In summary, our Creator, the Supreme Being whom most people call God, created everything and had set the rules for everything. We cannot separate our Creator from His creation, therefore, God is nature and nature is God. The rules that He had laid out to control everything is what we call, The Rules of Nature, or otherwise called the **Rules of God**. We cannot violate these rules; similarly, following these rules can only set us straight to our intended destination. So, to be healthy, to prevent illness as well as heal ourselves from ailments, then we should understand our bodies, how it functions and how to take care of it. We should try to minimize the use of all unnatural things and understand the Rules of Nature, follow it, and always remember the "Triad of Nature".

God created the world and the Universe in six days, and on the seventh day, He rested. These were God days which could mean many years per day. Today is still part of the seventh day, and God is still resting. God is not our servant plus He gave us the powers that we have now, tremendous powers, including the healing power. We should not only pray, but do what God wants us to do. That is to take care of each other, to love and respect each other and to value the human life. We have to remember that we are all "angels" to each other and that we all have "Divine Angels" watching over us.

So, what then is the role of acupuncture and traditional medicine in the treatment of illnesses? When an injury occurs, or an illness manifests, acupuncture should be the treatment of choice. In the absence of acupuncture, then energetic massage (EM) should be done. EM should be done as soon as possible and as often as possible while the illness or injury is still present. Medications should also be used concomitantly (or homeopathic medications) early on in order to provide comfort and rapid relief of symptoms. Medications used in the acute phase should not be used long term since they may cause problems like habituation or addiction. This is especially true for pain medications, specifically, narcotic pain medications. However, for long standing illnesses, then medications should be used to help the body recover while acupuncture and other complimentary treatments are being implemented, such as physical therapy, hypnosis, biofeedback, yoga, reflexology and other modalities. Medications alone should not be depended upon to correct a problem or illness. However, there will be situations wherein the use of medications or surgery is a must. But this should be done only after the patient has followed the habits of healthy living and the 10 Commandments of Health.

Finally, my final message is this, **"I don't seek perfection, I only seek for people to strive for perfection"**.

Henry Gacrama dela Torre, M.D., DABMA, FAAMA

ABOUT THE AUTHOR

Dr. Henry Gacrama dela Torre is a 1973 graduate of Cebu Institute of Medicine (Cebu City, Philippines) and trained in General Surgery at St. John's Episcopal Hospital in Brooklyn, New York. He started general practice in DuBois, Pennsylvania in December 1982. He is in the active medical staff of DuBois Regional Medical Center, DuBois, Pennsylvania. He studied Meridian Regulatory Acupuncture and Medical Hypnotherapy in the 1980s. In 2002, he finished the UCLA Helms Institute of Medical Acupuncture course, became board certified by the American Board of Medical Acupuncture in 2004, and became a Fellow of the American Academy of Medical Acupuncture in 2007. He also trained in Scalp Acupuncture, Korean Hand Therapy, and Five Elements Acupuncture.

BIBLIOGRAPHY

Acupuncture Energetics   Dr. Joseph Helms

The Foundations of Chinese Medicine   Giovanni Maciocia

Handbook of Chinese Herbal formula   Dr. Kris Yang

Textbook of General Medicine and Primary Care   Dr. John Noble

Principles of Internal Medicine 16th   Ed Harrison

Most of the concepts and the things I have written here are products of my own study, experience, observations, and application of the natural laws of physics. My acupuncture knowledge came mostly from the teachings of Dr. Joseph Helms and from Dr. Helm's book, Acupuncture Energetics.

ABOUT THE COVER

The cover of this book represents the relationship of God to nature and the relationship of things around us as provided to us by God. God breathe life to all the things that exist around us. He created the world and the universe for a reason. When God decided to put us on earth, He provided us with everything in order to survive. He created the sun as the center of life, the provider of energy to all living things on earth. It is said that man derives energy from the sun (Wei Qi) through our fingers (Ting points) and the energy circulates throughout our body and ultimately we are grounded to the earth through our feet (Ting points). This is a very important concept in acupuncture. In fact, this concept of being grounded to the earth is actually adopted by Clinton Ober, Dr. Stephen Sinatra and Martin Zucker in their book "Earthing". In the Five Element acupuncture, life started with the creation of the universe (including the sun). After the sun was created by God, He created the Earth. God then placed Metals inside the earth (mainly carbon) to help with its rotation, gravity and heating. Next, God placed the Oceans (Water) to complete the needs for life to exist. Then the trees were finally created by God to provide balance and nutrition to living things. I believe that God has used the "Rule of Three" in most things, including life itself. If we understand and maintain this relationship in nature, including our body, then there will be harmony and good health.

INDEX

A

abortion, spontaneous, 15
ACTH. *See* hormones: adrenocorticotropic
acupuncture, five element, 50, 52-53
acupuncture treatments, 111
adrenal burnout, 10
adrenaline, 75
Adrenocorticotrophic hormones, 2, 76
aldosterone, 75
Antidiuretic hormone, 76
Archangels, 1
astral body, 31, 88
Autonomic Nervous System, 72-74

B

basic elements, 50-51, 53
basis of energy, 37
basis of life, 37
bile, 18
biorhythm, 4, 6, 19
bladder channel, 6, 22, 82
  problems, 68
blood, functions of, 99
body
  channels of. *See* individual channels
  five senses of, 73
  reflexes of, gastrocolic, 7, 27
  systems of. *See* individual systems
  triads in, 109
body cavities, 23
body temperature, 21, 37, 88, 90, 99
brain needs, 5

C

carbohydrates, 100
cardiovascular system, 71, 79-80
cellular immunity, 17
Central Nervous System, 70, 72-73
chromosomal energy, 84. *See also* original energy
circulations in the body, 110
controlling cycle. *See* Ke Cycle
Controlling Energies, 10-11, 29-30
cortisol, 75
cycle of generation. *See* Sheng Cycle

D

dehydration, 87, 100, 109
detoxification, 6, 18, 24
diaphragm, 79-80
Diaphragmatic Fatigue Syndrome, 27
digestive system, 70, 77
diseases, 39, 102

dynamic energy, 30-31

E

Earth Element, 51
Electrostatic energy, 12
emotional factors, 16
endocrine system, 70, 74-75
energetic massage, 34, 44, 54, 69, 111
energetic personality, 14, 55, 62
energy
   nutritional. *See* Rong Qi
   original. *See* Yuan Qi
   protective. *See* Wei Qi
energy axes, 33
energy generation, 6, 6-7, 50
energy pool, 11, 30
energy production, 37
essence of life, 23, 84
essentials to life, 110
excretory system, 71, 81
external devils (dragons), 16

F

Fire Element, 51
flash signs, 67
flow of nutritional energy, 19-26
follicle stimulating hormone, 76
forces that affect the pregnancy, 16

G

gallbladder channel, 6, 23
   problems, 68
gastrocolic reflex, 27
gastroesophageal reflux disease, 27
Genetic Energy, 9, 13-14, 45, 98. *See also* original energy
genetic impurities, 15
genetic problems, 14

glucagon, 75, 78
growth hormone, 76

H

hair, 93
headaches, 25, 31
healing, essentials, 110
healing triad, 34
health, 6, 117
   maintenance of, 25, 110
   problems for, 108
   ten commandments of, 103
heart, 17, 21-22, 79-81
   functions, 110
heart channel, 6, 20-21, 71
   problems, 68
heater
   lower, 23
   middle, 23
   upper, 23
heating triad, 38
Hematologic System, 71, 87
homosexuality, factors causing, 97
hormones
   adrenal, 7
      adrenaline, 2, 4, 7-8, 18, 76, 87
      aldosterone, 76
      cortisol, 4, 7, 18, 75-76
   adrenomedullary, 4
   growth, 76
humoral immunity, 17

I

immune system, 86
Indirect Wei Qi, 30
insulin, 20, 75
Integumentary System, 71, 88
internal devils (dragons), 16
involuntary functions, 17

J

Jing, 23, 84-85, 104
Jue Yin, 34
Jue Yin Fire, 56, 61
Jue Yin Wood, 56, 60

K

Ke Cycle, 51-53
kidney channel, 8, 17-18, 22, 81
   problems, 67
kidneys, functions of, 90-91

L

large intestine channel, 6-7, 23, 27
   problems, 68
law of deficiency and excesses, 108
life, 37-39, 116-17
   essence of, 23, 84
   essentials to, 110
   source of, 79
Life essence, 104
liver, functions, 10, 18-19, 23-24, 29, 34, 36, 45, 50, 54, 65, 72, 74, 77-78, 82, 88, 105-6
liver channel, 6, 18, 24, 83
   problems, 68
lung channel, 7, 26
   problems, 68

M

massage, energetic, 44, 111-12, 114
master of the heart channel, 23, 45
maximum functional time, 5
melatonin, 2, 76
metabolism, 2, 43, 45, 78
Metal Element, 7, 51, 53
mind, 23, 56, 63-64, 104
Motor Nervous System, 73
muscle spasm, triad, 83
musculoskeletal system, 71, 83

N

nature's triad (dela Torre Triad), 110
nervous system, 18
Nutrition
   primary, 110
   secondary, 110
Nutritional Energy, 2, 5, 7, 9-11, 16-17, 19-20, 23-24, 29-31, 33, 45, 71, 97

O

obstructive sleep apnea, 27
Original Energy, 10, 13-14, 84, 96-98
overall planning of the body's functions, 78. *See also* liver
oxygen, 37-38, 99

P

pancreas, 78
parathyroid gland, 75
Parathyroid hormone, 75
personality, product of, 14
pituitary gland, 17
Premature balding, graying, 23
Protective energy, 2, 11-12, 30, 98, 111
protein, 37

R

radiation, 29
renin, 75
reproductive system, 84-86
respiratory system, 70, 78

resting period, 5
Rong Qi, 2, 17-20, 25, 27

S

Sensory Nervous System, 73
sexual activity, 84-86, 95, 98
Shao Yang, 33, 56, 61
Shao Yang Fire, 56, 62
Shao Yang Wood, 56, 62
Shao Yin, 33, 36, 55, 57
Shao Yin Fire, 55, 57
Shao Yin Water, 55, 57
Sheng Cycle, 50-52
sins against the body and nature, 105
sins of modern society, 28
small intestine channel, 6, 22
  problems, 68
soul, 63-66, 104, 116
Soul, 63-66
Spirit, structural foundation, 104
spleen channel, 18, 20
  problems, 68
spontaneous abortion, 15
Steal Syndrome, 20
stem cells, 9
stomach channel, 6-7, 19, 27
  problems, 68
storage of blood, 78, 99
stored energy, 30
Structural Biopsychotypes, 55, 57
sun, 2, 4, 25, 29, 32, 88-89, 116
sunlight, 2

T

Tai Yang, 33, 55-56
Tai Yang Fire, 55-56
Tai Yang Water, 55-56
Tai Yin, 34, 36, 55, 58
Tai Yin Earth, 55, 58
Tai Yin Metal, 55, 58

Ten Commandments of Health, 69, 102-3
thyroid gland, 46
thyroid stimulating hormone, 76
ting points, 94, 125
triad, 108-10
triad of healing, 108
triple heater channel, 6, 19, 23, 33-34, 51, 54, 72
triple warmer. *See* triple heater channel

V

vitamin D, 2, 32, 84, 88
voluntary functions, 17

W

water, 38-39, 99
water balance, 82, 99
Water Element, 51
Wei Qi, 2, 32
wood element, 50, 53
Wood Element, 53

Y

yang, 37, 50, 54, 82
yang astral body, 31
yang excess syndrome, 40, 43-44, 47
Yang Ming, 34, 36, 56
Yang Ming Earth, 56
Yang Ming Metal, 56, 59
yin, 38-39, 82
yin astral body, 31
yin deficiency syndrome, 40, 45, 47
youthful look, 104
Yuan Qi, 9-16
yuan Qi, growth and development of the fetus, 14
Yuan Qi, *See also* Jing

www.ingramcontent.com/pod-product-compliance
Lightning Source LLC
Chambersburg PA
CBHW021956170526
45157CB00003B/1022